Children on Medication Volume II

Epilepsy, Emotional Disturbance, and Adolescent Disorders

Kenneth D. Gadow, Ph.D.
Department of Psychiatry
State University of New York
at Stony Brook

Taylor & Francis
London and Philadelphia

Published by
Taylor & Francis Ltd, 4 John Street, London WC1N 2ET

First published by College-Hill Press, San Diego, California

British Library Cataloguing in Publication Data

This edition not for sale in the American continent.

0850666333

Printed in the United States of America

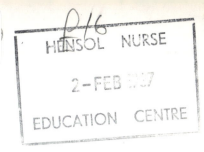
Children on Medication II

Dedicated to the teachers, parents, and children who, by their participation in medical and psychological research, have made this book possible. Their unselfish support of clinical research will allow subsequent generations to reap the benefits of scientific inquiry, just as we all benefit from the efforts of those who have preceded us.

CONTENTS

FOREWORD

One of the most notable aspects about the topic of this book is the vast gaps in some areas of knowledge. Often these vast gaps in knowledge are in extremely important areas. The author cites several examples to illustrate the point being made. For example, in the chapter entitled "Seizure Disorders: Early Childhood and Mental Retardation," he notes that "there have been few published accounts about how to improve the way in which pharmacotherapy is typically managed" (p. 92). A similar gap exists in regard to available information for educators, including teachers, special education teachers, supervisors, and principals, as well as for parents. Fortunately, this situation is being greatly reduced by the publication of the second edition of *Children on Medication*.

Another example of a glaring gap in the clinical data base pertains to information about reducing and terminating psychotropic medication. To put this in perspective, consider that there are probably 750 articles in the medical literature describing how to use psychotropic medication (usually stimulants for hyperactive children), but probably fewer than 10 articles that address explicitly how to either reduce or terminate medication for a child who no longer needs it (Reatig, 1984). Surely this is an unbalanced and one-sided approach to say the least. This book seeks to remedy such one-sided approaches.

Before leaving this topic, a few comments are in order about how this situation arose in the first place. There really is no evidence in medical literature that explains why there are glaring gaps in knowledge that have not been addressed by scholars or researchers, but it seems that the most likely explanation is the philosophical orientation of the medical scholars and researchers who write in this area. The primary orientation of these writers is the biomedical model which emphasizes biological etiology (causes) and medical interventions (treatments), in this case, psychotropic medication. Keep in mind that the biomedical model has been, fortunately for the welfare of mankind, quite successful in many acute biological disorders; the ancient scourge of mankind, smallpox, has now been eliminated from the world largely due to following techniques outlined by the biomedical model. In spite of such notable feats, the biomedical model is much less helpful in chronic disorders that are influenced by educational, behavioral, and sociological factors. Areas of high interest to parents and educators are often considered outside the purview of the biomedical model, thus such problems are all too often ignored by researchers.

Anyone with a chronic medical problem in the family quickly realizes how important it is to have readable, accurate, and nontechnical sources of information about the chronic disease of importance to them. At this point I am not writing about an abstract idea that seems valid on the basis of my reading and research, but I am describing a week-after-week situation in my own family involving kidney failure, a serious chronic medical disorder, in which pertinent, readable information is very important, sometimes involving life-or-death types of decisions. As many others have found to be the case, the printed material supplied by well-meaning staff members simply does not satisfy the information needs of a paient's family. In this context, it is with considerable pleasure that I write this preface and state that this edition fills a very important glaring gap in the psychopharmacological literature. In appropriately detailed fashion, with the introduction of technical terms and subsequent defintions only when needed, the edition oovors a broad range of issues surrounding the often controversial question of administering medication to an exceptional child or adolescent.

Finally, as an instructor of a university course on psychotropic medication in children for the past 17 years, I certainly look forward to the appearance of this edition to use as a textbook for special education students who enroll and who are often bewildered by the mass of technical information that is available in the medical literature on the topic. So, for these prospective students and the families of the exceptional children receiving psychotropic medication, I endorse this volume for those seeking information about such medication use in children and adolescents.

REFERENCE

Reatig, N. (1984). Attention deficit disorder: A bibliography. *Psychopharmacology Bulletin, 20,* 693–730.

ROBERT L. SPRAGUE, Ph.D.

FOREWORD

In almost every school program that addresses the behavioral and educational needs of children, the topic of medication is at some time discussed. Be it from an anxious parent, teacher, administrator, or other caregiver, the topic remains a highly volatile one often open to many interpretations.

For years, teachers and other caregivers have been kept in the dark concerning the use of medications prescribed to their children. This situation has often led to a mystifying reliance on those who have prescribed the medications. In many ways this lack of information was used to excuse acceptable and valid reasons for inappropriate behavior or academic difficulties. By removing or at least clarifying the medication mystic, Gadow, in this book, attempts to provide for the first time critical information that is sorely lacking.

It is especially important to note that Gadow does not attempt to make everyone who reads this book into medical practitioners. He is quick to point out that his major goal is to provide much-needed pharmacological information that will help caregivers better understand medical decisions. This is especially important today in light of societies' growing obsession with drugs and their side effects.

Gadow clearly points out that important pharmacological work has been published in the past, but for *select* professional populations. This landmark attempt, however, puts all related and needed information together in a single resource to be read and referred to by diverse populations of professional and lay people.

Finally, Gadow, in what I have come to know as his typically thorough and persevering style, and in his effort to teach us as much as possible, has developed a suggested reading list and glossary that acts as an aid in clarifying fundamental medication concepts and terms.

In summary, this book is both a technically detailed resource and a reference guide. It is clearly written and succinctly outlines the path the reader is to take as he or she approaches different disability areas or child domains. In many ways this resource is unique in that it addresses the needs of a professional audience as well as those parents who for years have been left with unanswered pharmacological questions. Gadow's discussion of psychotropic drugs, how physicians prescribe drugs in everyday situations, and the timely discussion of trade versus generic names are but some examples that prove to be especially helpful.

Having been on the administrative and teaching side of working with handicapped children for almost two decades, and having had the opportunity to review Dr. Gadow's work, I can unequivocally say that those working with handicapped children now have a comprehensive resource to which they can turn much in the same way as the physician has had his or her desk reference (PDR).

As with most comprehensive resources, time will dictate how well this book is received. Personally, I have already found it to be invaluable.

Michael Bender, Ed.D.

ACKNOWLEDGMENTS

This book was made possible through the efforts of many people. The author would like to express appreciation to the following people for making prepublication materials, copyrighted figures and tables, or lengthy quotations available to me: Magda Campbell, John Kalachnik, Samuel Livingston, Esther Sleator, and Robert Sprague. I would like to thank Dr. John Pomeroy, former Chief of Child Psychiatry Service at the State University of New York at Stony Brook, for preparing a most informative chapter on adolescent psychiatric disorders for this volume. I am also most grateful to Lucinda Lindgren and Gretchen Daly for their role in helping to prepare various drafts of manuscript.

I am very grateful to the literally hundreds of teachers and parents in Illinois who supplied the necessary information to describe therapeutic drug use patterns among children in special education programs and to the Directors of Special Education, school administrators, and school nurses who made these data collection efforts possible. A special thanks is extended to my interviewers, Jan Knecht, Tobey Fumento, and Norma Wilson.

I wish especially to express appreciation to my colleagues at the Institute for Child Behavior and Development (University of Illinois ar Urbana-Champaign), particularly Robert L. Sprague and Esther Sleator, for their encouragement and support over the years. They provided a most unique environment in which to learn about pediatric psychopharmacotherapy; one that emphasized both methodological rigor and clinical common sense.

Introduction

The primary purpose of this book is to provide information about the use of medication for a variety of childhood disorders that require long-term treatment. It is the author's expectation that this information will allow caregivers to make better decisions about the use of pharmacotherapy. Unfortunately, knowing what to do is often not a simple matter of right versus wrong or correct versus incorrect but rather the product of a complex set of evaluations pertaining to the characteristics of the child and the family and school setting. Before addressing the text's role with regard to this process, it is important to explain exactly what kinds of drugs and disorders are discussed here.

Among the most commonly prescribed drugs for children that are administered on a long-term basis are the psychotropics and the antiepileptics. *Psychotropic* drugs are generally prescribed to control mood, thought processes, and behavior. These drugs are familiar to most of us and include the following: stimulants, antidepressants, neuroleptics (major tranquilizers), antianxiety agents (minor tranquilizers), hypnotics, and sedatives. In children they are prescribed for a variety of disorders, such as hyperactivity, aggression, nocturnal enuresis (bed wetting), anxiety, sleep problems, and so forth. *Antiepileptic* drugs are generally prescribed for seizure disorders, but they do have other applications. Together, these two groups of drugs account for much, but certainly not all, of the medication prescribed for children and adolescents.

Early in my experiences with children in special education programs, it became evident that medications and the disorders for which they were prescribed affected the lives of many people, often in very important ways. Yet there was little opportunity for caregivers to learn about drugs, their intended therapeutic effects, and their unwanted side effects. Moreover, the information that was available was often inaccurate or incomplete (e.g., in the child's school medical records) or too technical for lay audiences (e.g., in a medical reference book). In recent years there have been numerous attempts to fill this void, a fact that can be readily confirmed by a casual perusal of the paperback books placed in the health care section of your local bookstore.

Although it might be inferred from this observation that the information problem has been addressed, it is my impression that many texts aimed at lay audiences are too superficial, incomplete with regard to treatment practices and controversies and silent on the topic of the psychosocial aspects of pharmacotherapy. What is really needed is a technically detailed reference that is both readable and to the point. It should be thorough enough to be useful for medical personnel who have limited experience in this area (but who are nevertheless called upon to manage such cases after the specialist initiates treatment) and yet free of medical jargon so the lay person can appreciate the factual content. It should strive to focus on clinical management and refrain from speculating about the implications of laboratory findings that are loosely connected to real world situations. Moreover, it is probably fair to say that although much of our research efforts generates greater understanding of these children, their problems, and their reaction to medication, on a year-to-year basis, very few studies actually effect changes in treatment practices for a particular disorder. In fact, since the first edition of this book was published, very few "new" drugs (or new applications for existing drugs) have appeared on the scene (see, for example, Campbell et al., 1983, and Gualtieri et al., 1983).

The use of drug therapy in the management of childhood psychiatric disorders and to some extent seizure disorders has received much attention in recent years. One can walk into almost any public school, special education facility, residential placement, sheltered workshop, or community-based program for the handicapped and, after engaging teachers and staff in a conversation about children and medication, discover that this is quite a controversial topic. Such discussions not only reveal a considerable interest in medication but also a variety of problems associated with drug threapy (see, for example, Gadow, 1982a). Unfortunately, it is difficult for people outside the medical professions to learn about the therapeutic use of psychotropic and antiepileptic drugs. It is not unusual, therefore, that many caregivers are poorly informed about medication. This lack of knowledge is often accompanied by uncertainties and misconceptions that are created, in part, by sensational articles in popular periodicals and newspapers. The fact that researchers and clinicians simply do not know all the answers to frequently asked questions about pharmacotherapy also complicates matters. Highly biased articles both for and against drug treatment have fueled a bitter controversy over the use of medication for certain childhood disorders. Because little is known about the etiology (causes) of most of these maladies, a number of prophets have surfaced willing to lead us to the truth. In the center of this confusion, controversy, and uncertainty are the family, school, and health care providers trying to figure out what is the best thing to do for their children, and they are not always in agreement.

WHY LEARN ABOUT DRUG TREATMENT?

The use of medication in the management of behavior and seizure disorders is of interest to caregivers for several reasons:

1. The very behaviors that are altered by drugs are often interrelated with the educational, habilitative, and parenting process. For example, severe behavior disorders can interfere with the child's ability to benefit from instruction as well as hinder the teacher's efforts to teach other children in the class. Physically aggressive acts can actually place the welfare of both caregiver and peers in jeopardy. Similarly, uncontrolled seizures can be a serious impediment to learning for the child with epilepsy. If the attacks are frequent or severe, the amount of time spent on instruction can be greatly limited. Seizures in the classroom or in recreational and neighborhood settings can be quite disruptive for peers as well if the situation is not handled appropriately. Because these chronic childhood conditions often precipitate serious emotional problems, caregivers can become involved in another aspect of child development: social adjustment. One way severe behavior disorders become a part of the teaching process is when they are identified as instructional objectives. This is particularly true in special education settings.
2. Medication is of interest to caregivers because the drugs used in the management of these disorders may have a pronounced effect on behavior. In some children, medication suppresses behavior that is perceived as incompatible with accepted standards. For other children, drug therapy appears to make then more responsive to their environment by enhancing cognitive abilities. Also of importance are the adverse effects of medication. Although many side effects are benign or eventually go away, others can be quite alarming if those responsible for the

child's care are unprepared for what to expect. When side effects impair adaptive behavior (e.g., learning ability, social interaction) or create emotional problems, they are not only distressing to caregivers but raise serious risk-to-benefit questions.

3. Studies have shown that relatively large numbers of school-aged children in special education programs are on medication for epilepsy and severe behavior disorders (Gadow, 1981, 1982b). In fact, few child care providers have not had some experience with youngsters who were receiving medication for one of these maladies. Pharmacotherapy is particularly common for children in special education programs for the mentally retarded and emotionally disturbed (behavior disordered).

4. Studies have clearly demonstrated the importance of feedback from caregivers in making treatment-related decisions (Sprague & Gadow, 1976). Teachers, for example, can be helpful by providing the child's physician with behavioral evaluations during the diagnostic, dosage adjustment, and followup phases of drug treatment. Reports of side effects observed in the home, classroom, or community setting are also valuable. Because medication does not teach the child anything, many children with learning and behavior problems will require educational or habilitative programming as part of the total treatment plan. It has been my experience that caregivers are often very interested in therapeutic measures that have an impact upon their own efforts. Charles Bradley (1957), one of the important historical figures in pediatric psychopharmacology, expressed his thoughts on the matter as follows:

> It is probably helpful for the teacher to have some understanding of the effect any medication may be having on the child's behavior. Teachers as well as parents can be more objective when they understand the true nature of a child's difficulty, and the physician may often wisely make the proper interpretation to them if the parents so desire. (p. 1058)

OBJECTIVES OF THIS BOOK

After conducting three statewide studies about how medication was being used with children in special education programs, I realized that teachers and parents were interested in drug treatment and were concerned about a number of treatment-related problems. Perhaps the greatest single problem is a lack of information about drug therapy. Caregivers have many questions about what medication is supposed to do to help children, side effects, whether drugs can interfere with learning, dosage, what people should do in various treatment-related situations, drug interactions, and what kinds of drugs are used for specific disorders (Gadow, 1982a).

Because there are few comprehensive references for parents, teachers, and health care providers about drug therapy, this book was developed to answer these and other questions about children on medication. It must be emphasized that making drug information available in this format does not imply that nonmedical caregivers should preempt a medical role! School personnel, for example, should not make medical diagnoses or recommend to parents that their child should be placed on medication. It is generally agreed, however, that teachers can be helpful to physicians by providing much needed feedback about the response to treatment. The school is but a part of a team effort that involves the family, health professions, psychological services, and social welfare agencies. It is hoped that by making drug information available to parents and nonmedical professionals, they will be more effective in participating in an interdisciplinary treatment effort.

The primary focus of this book is a description of the behavioral effects of drugs and the primary side effects observable to caregivers. Although questions are frequently asked about how medication acts on the body to produce certain behavioral changes, this topic is not discussed here. A lack of understanding on the part of the reader about how a drug works should not interfere in any way with the expressed objectives of this text.

There is always a danger, of course, that a frank discussion of adverse drug reactions may deter parents from obtaining desirable and quite possibly necessary treatment. The reader must bear in mind that almost all forms of therapy are associated with some risk. These risks, moreover, may very well be less serious that the consequences of ignoring true therapeutic needs. It should also be emphasized that many psychotropic and antiepileptic drugs are true miracles of modern pharmacological research. Their role in reducing human pain and suffering can be readily confirmed by simply reading about or talking with someone who is familiar with the situation that existed in our mental health facilities prior to the mid 1950s. Side effects information is provided here not to alarm caregivers but rather to prepare them for their possible occurrence and in so doing alleviate the intense anxiety associated with unexpected drug-related phenomena. Fortunately, the majority of commonly prescribed psychotropic and antiepileptic drugs are associated with low levels of risk when used and monitored appropriately.

Of equal importance to discussing drug-related changes in behavior is describing how doctors use medication. This includes typical dosages, the time of day medication is taken, how long treatment will last, and under what circumstances medication is terminated. This is much more difficult than it sounds because few people study the behavior of physicians (or teachers or other professionals for that matter). Although there are many statements of clinical experience in the literature or "how to treat" articles, there is often a disparity between what experts say should be done and what really happens in everyday situations. In order to create a more realistic picture of actual practices, the available data on everyday medical procedures are included.

The effective use of medical technology is an art. Physicians, like most professionals, develop a variety of ways for handling similar problems based upon the responses of previous patients. The reader is cautioned, therefore, that the descriptions of medical practices presented in this text are not necessarily what might be encountered or what should necessarily be expected. Many people are uncomfortable with this underlying degree of uncertainty that characterizes psychotropic drug therapy for childhood and adolescent disorders. It is, nevertheless, a reality and we should all recognize the limitations of medical science. Gualtieri et al. (1983) have described this situation as follows:

> Diagnosis and prediction of drug response are not exact sciences. The child, treated with a psychoactive agent, is in reality a research subject. The only real measure of good practice is an empirical approach to the individual child. Management of difficult behaviors by the administration of psychotropic drugs is justifiable only in the context of an individualized and comprehensive therapeutic program. (p. 202)

WHAT'S MISSING

There is a point after which detail becomes either impractical or counterproductive, and subsequently decisions had to be made with regard to which topics were going to be briefly cited or omitted altogether. In this text, the following question aided in making this decision: Does an understanding of this topic provide insight into how a particular disorder should (or is) generally managed? Among the topics that have received more limited treatment are etiology (causes), diagnostic procedures, and neuropharmacology (how drugs affect the nervous system). The necessary focus on medical intervention has precluded any explanation of the social-emotional problems associated with chronic childhood disorders. It is hoped that this will not obscure the importance of *psychosocial* factors in the etiology, response to treatment, and long-term therapeutic outcome of behavior and seizure disorders. What may to some be a limitation is the secondary treatment of alternative therapeutic procedures. It would be truly unfortunate to infer from this decision that drug therapy is the sole treatment for severe behavior disorders and epilepsy or even the best method for all or most children with psychiatric disorders. Because many books and articles are available about nonmedical techniques, it seemed unnecessary to review them in any detail here. Instead, publications discussing alternative measures are cited as references.

TRADE NAMES VERSUS GENERIC NAMES

If for no other reason than a financial one, most people are aware of the fact that drugs possess both trade names and generic names. In general, if a particular medicine is available in both trade and generic forms, the latter is less expensive. A *trade name* is a registered trademark, and only the holder of the trademark or its legal representative can ever use the trade name to sell medicine. A *generic name* is a scientific name that is recognized throughout the world and is used by scientists and clinicians in scientific papers and textbooks.

To more fully understand the significance of the differences between these two terms, the reader should also know that a drug manufacturer typically patents a newly formulated agent and controls the rights to manufacture it for 17 years. This time period is provided, in part, to allow the drug company an opportunity to recoup its financial investment into the product. In reality, however, it usually takes several years to obtain Food and Drug Administration (FDA) approval to market a new drug in the United States, so the actual period of competition-free merchandising is actually much shorter. During this competition-free period, the drug company seeks to establish brand loyalty through the use of its trade name. In other words, after the patent has expired, many clinicians will continue to write prescriptions for the trade name. To help insure this response, drugs were often given complicated generic names that were difficult to spell and remember. For example, the generic name for Ritalin is methylphenidate hydrochloride. Obviously, it is much easier to write and remember the word Ritalin. This situation changed, due in part to the passage of the 1962 Kefauver-Harris Amendments to the Food, Drug, and Cosmetic Act of 1938. Following the passage of this legislation, the United States Adopted Names Council, which is supervised by the federal government, was established to decide whether or not a generic name is suitable (Silverman & Lee, 1974, p. 37).

The importance of these facts is that when the period of patent protection expires, any drug company can then manufacture the drug and sell it either by its generic name or by a different trade name. The generic drug manufacturer profits by selling the drug in large volume at a lower price. There has been, and continues to be, a considerable debate concerning generic drugs. The primary issue has been the question of *bioavailability*. It has been alleged that certain generic drugs may not be identical to the trade name product because they do not reach and concentrate in the same body areas as the trade name product to a comparable degree. Some have even argued that generic products should undergo the same exact intense scrutiny by the FDA as new drugs.

This somewhat detailed discussion of generic and trade names is presented here for more than just educational purposes. It is also intended to help explain why trade names are used in this text and why this will be viewed as unacceptable by some. It could be said that, in view of the aforementioned discussion, the use of trade names in a textbook constitutes a form of advertising for a particular product. The justification for using trade names here is threefold. One, most psychotropic and antiepileptic drug prescriptions for children are still written for trade name products. Therefore, caregivers generally encounter trade names. Two, generic drug products are not necessarily available, even if the period of patent protection has expired. And three, a careful examination of the research on the topics addressed in this book will show that most studies acknowledge that the drug or drugs employed were supplied by the trade name manufacturer. In a certain sense, our scientific knowledge is based upon trade name products. Although this explanation will not satisfy everyone, the purpose of this text is to provide drug information to help people who are not medically trained in the use of a particular drug to make better treatment-related decisions. Suffice it to say, then, that the scientific literature generally uses generic names and that generic products, if available, will probably be less expensive than trade name products. For those who are more familiar with generic names, conversion from trade to generic name can be achieved quite easily by simply referring to Appendix D.

INTERNATIONAL AUDIENCE

This book has been prepared with the intent of reaching an international audience interested in the pharmacological management of child and adolescent disorders. Two steps have been taken in an attempt to achieve this goal. One has been the formulation of a special list of trade names and their associated generic names for *some* products marketed in the United Kingdom and Western Europe (see Appendix H). The formulation of an exhaustive list is an almost insurmountable task because there are no consistent rules for trade name use. The problem is compounded by the fact that there are hundreds of psychotropic and antiepileptic drugs and an even greater number of countries. As was previously discussed, Appendix D can be used to resolve any confusion concerning a specific trade name.

The second step toward an international approach has been the inclusion of research and discussions of clinical practice from scientists and clinicians throughout the world. It is important to emphasize that there are often major differences of opinion from one country to the next on how medication should be used.

Reaching an international audience is made more difficult by the fact that (a) generic names are not always identical and (b) the rules for conducting research and obtaining governmental approval for the use of new agents vary greatly, so it is possible for a particular drug to be popularly used in one country and not yet available in another. The first problem, internationally inconsistent generic names, can be either minor or major depending upon the drug. For example, the drug known as phenobarbital in the United States was referred to as phenobarbitone in the United Kingdom, a difference that would be of trivial consequence. However, the antiepileptic drug known as valproic acid (Depakene) in the United States is referred to as sodium valproate (Epilim) in the United Kingdom. This example is of course much more problematical. Interestingly, the actual chemical formulation of these two products differs slightly, hence the different generic names. The second problem, differential government regulation procedures, is more difficult to resolve. Basically, with few exceptions, the drugs discussed in this book are only those that are approved for use in the United States.

SUGGESTED READINGS

Given the varied background of the intended audience and its equally diverse information needs, each chapter includes a list of suggested readings for those interested in pursuing a particular topic in greater detail. It has been my experience that it is very difficult to find a "good" article on a specific medical topic without knowing someone who is trained in that area. The suggested readings listed in this text are ones that may be particularly useful for more extensive study. These are not, however, exhaustive lists, and the failure to cite a particular reference should not be misconstrued as judgmental. The existing medical literature is so staggering (see Durack, 1978) that it was possible to cite only a few representative examples for each area. Each item in the list is coded for the audience for which it is most appropriate: P = parent, S = school personnel, and C = clinician. Many items in the last category are suitable for graduate students in the behavioral sciences. Because this book was designed to serve as an introduction to the medical literature, many of the sources cited as being appropriate for clinicians are also suitable for motivated parents and school personnel. Fortunately, the prudent course of action in many treatment-related situations is nothing more than common sense, provided that there is access to all relevant information.

GLOSSARY

The demystification of scientific areas can often be achieved by simply adopting nontechnical terminology to explain fundamental concepts. This is successful in many instances, but in others it makes more sense to define and subsequently use the scientific term. This book employs both approaches. Although the decision to use a particular technical term may appear to be arbitrary, the author has attempted to select and use those which were deemed useful for interdisciplinary collaboration and further study. A glossary of terms appears at the back of the book to assist the reader in deciphering medically oriented discussions of drug therapy. Each term is defined in nontechnical language, and the reader is encouraged to refer to it whenever necessary. The glossary should help solve the problem of terms that are defined in earlier chapters of the text, but which are encountered for the first time by readers who select particular topics for reference purposes.

COMPANION VOLUMES

The first edition of *Children on Medication* attempted to present an overview of pediatric psychopharmacology in one volume. As the current revision progressed, however, with its expanded range of topics and increased depth of detail, it soon became apparent that a single volume was no longer feasible, practical, or desirable. For example, one of the major impediments to acquiring medical information is an economic one. Most medical references are simply too expensive for the average reader. True, although some are available in public libraries, their treatment of medication for specific conditions is often greatly limited by their expressed need to discuss a variety of disorders. Rather than add another expensive text to the list of available medical reference books, it was decided to divide *Children on Medication* into companion volumes. This not only allowed a closer approximation of the goal of economic feasibility but also provided the reader with an opportunity to select topics of greatest interest. Fortunately, the content lent itself to such a division, and two separate books were formulated, one subtitled *Hyperactivity, Learning Disabilities, and Mental Retardation* and a second subtitled *Epilepsy, Emotional Disturbance, and Adolescent Disorders*. The goal was to formulate two volumes that would be fairly equivalent in price to one large book.

In creating two volumes of *Children on Medication*, it was necessary to repeat some material such as the Appendices and the Glossary. The first chapter, "Fundamental Concepts in Pharmacotherapy: An Overview," is an abridged version of the chapter that appears in the companion volume. The abridged chapter was included in the present book so that it could stand on its own as a complete text. It was also necessary to resist the temptation to make the discussion of each disorder even more comprehensive by adding peripheral but related topics, because this obviously would have only resulted in the recurrence of the initial problem.

ORGANIZATION OF THE BOOK

This book, *Epilepsy, Emotional Disturbance, and Adolescent Disorders*, describes antiepileptic drug therapy for epilepsy (seizure disorders), childhood psychoses such as infantile autism and schizophrenia, a variety of adolescent psychiatric disorders (e.g., schizophrenia and depression), and several miscellaneous conditions, such as enuresis and cerebral palsy, that are difficult to group under a particular heading. Many, but certainly not all, of these disorders share the characteristics of being (a) relatively low prevalence disabilities (at least when compared with hyperactivity, learning disability, and mental retardation), (b) more commonly recognized as organically based, particularly seizure disorders and severe emotional disturbance, and (c) more readily accepted as medical conditions by the general public.

The companion volume, *Hyperactivity, Learning Disabilities, and Mental Retardation*, focuses primarily on psychotropic drug use for hyperactivity and aggressiveness, two disorders that often co-occur. Because academic underachievement is often, but certainly not always, an associated problem, it seemed logical to include these three disorders in the same text. A separate chapter appears on mental retardation because hyperactive behavior and aggressiveness is often managed in very different ways for children and adolescents who are mentally retarded compared with their nonretarded peers. This is especially true for mentally retarded people who live in institutional settings and for those who are more severely retarded.

The general outline of each book is as follows: Chapter 1 explains some of the fundamental concepts and terms relating to drug therapy. Each of the following chapters covers the use of medication with regard to specific childhood disorders. However, their arrangement is somewhat different from most medical texts on medication. Instead of grouping the topics by psychiatric diagnoses, more functional categories were used both from the standpoint of drug therapy and from the caregiver's frame of reference. Three categorical systems were used to formulate the two medical volumes: diagnosis, special education, and age. Two of the more common medical disorders for which drugs are prescribed (hyperactivity and seizure disorders) are discussed in some detail, a separate chapter for each. There are also separate chapters for three of the major (on the basis of prevalence) handicapping conditions recognized by special education professionals (learning disabilities, emotional disturbance, and mental retardation). This seemed prudent given the relatively high rates of drug use among children and adolescents in these programs (e.g., Epstein et al., 1985; Gadow, 1981; Safer & Krager, 1984). Moreover, parents and, of course, school personnel are more inclined to think of children in terms of special education categorical labels. The third categorical system is represented here with separate chapters about preschool-aged children and adolescents. Middle childhood is the primary focus of the other chapters. To facilitate pursuit of a particular disorder, careful attention has been given to the Subject Index, and many topics are cross-referenced within the text.

When available, prevalence figures are reported for each disorder and for the use of drug therapy in the general school population and in special education programs. Both therapeutic effects and side effects of the drugs employed are described, along with the pattern of treatment. The latter includes dosage, schedule of drug administration, duration of treatment, and drug combinations. Because drugs typically have many pharmacological properties, they are often used in the management of more than one disorder. To prevent the redundancy that would result from describing the same drug in different chapters, only the primary drugs associated with the treatment of each condition are discussed in any detail.

To repeat, by no means should the intent of these books be misconstrued as implying that school personnel, parents, or other nonmedical personnel should assume the role of a physician. However, if it enabled caregivers to ask more intelligent questions during interdisciplinary interaction and to focus more clearly on educational and child development issues, then these texts will have fulfilled their purpose. It is hoped one byproduct of this increased awareness will be a more satisfactory life experience for the child, the true objective of our efforts as parents, educators, and clinicians.

Epilepsy, Emotional Disturbance, and Adolescent Disorders

Chapter 1: Fundamental Concepts in Pharmacotherapy: An Overview. The first chapter presents a brief introduction to the different kinds of drugs that are used to effect changes in mood, thought processes, and behavior and an overview of some basic concepts in drug therapy such as dosage adjustment, tolerance, and side effects.

Chapter 2: Seizure Disorders. There are a number of seizure disorders, and they differ from one another in terms of what the seizures look like, age when attacks usually begin, and type of drug that is most effective in controlling the seizures. The main focus of this chapter is a description of the various types of epilepsy and the drugs used to treat them. Other topics include febrile seizures, the management of seizures in the classroom, the circumstances under which drug treatment is terminated, and how antiepileptic drugs can affect classroom performance. Because many children who have a seizure disorder receive two or more drugs per day, drug interactions are also discussed.

Chapter 3: Seizure Disorders: Early Childhood and Mental Retardation. Antiepileptic drug therapy is particularly common among children in two special education categories, early childhood and mental retardation. This chapter addresses the special problems seizure disorders present for these two populations of children and their clinical implications.

Chapter 4: Emotional Disturbance. Unquestionably, two of the most disabling childhood disorders for which psychotropic drugs may be prescribed are infantile autism and childhood schizophrenia. At the present time, the neuroleptics appear to be the drugs of choice for children for whom this treatment is appropriate. Two additional childhood disorders for which the term *emotional disturbance* could be considered appropriate, at least as it is used by the special education community, are childhood depression and conduct disorder. This chapter discusses drug treatment for each of these disorders and presents a special overview of neuroleptic drug use for preschool-aged autistic children.

Chapter 5: Adolescent Psychiatric Disorders. This chapter addresses the use of psychotropic drugs for the treatment of adolescent psychiatric disorders. They are grouped here according to areas of functioning: mood (mania, depression), thinking (psychosis), conduct (aggression, hyperactivity), eating (anorexia nervosa, bulimia, obesity), and emotions (anxiety, phobias, and obsessional disorders). Although the most suitable drugs for the management of these disorders vary depending upon the condition being treated, two broad groups of drugs, the neuroleptics and antidepressants, are the primary focus of this discussion. Special attention has been given to the behavioral characteristics of each disorder.

Chapter 6: Other Disorders. The final chapter briefly describes the use of psychotropic drugs for enuresis (bedwetting), school phobia (separation anxiety), cerebral palsy, and Tourette syndrome. The tricyclic antidepressants (e.g., Tofranil) have been used with some success in the treatment of enuresis and school phobia. The two most commonly prescribed skeletal muscle relaxants for cerebral palsy are Valium and Dantrium. A variety of drugs have been used to treat Tourette syndrome, but the neuroleptics are generally considered the most effective agents at the present time.

Hyperactivity, Learning Disabilities, and Mental Retardation

Chapter 1: Fundamental Concepts in Pharmacotherapy. The first chapter is a brief introduction to the different kinds of drugs that are used to effect changes in mood, thought processes, and behavior. Central to an appreciation for the complexity of drug treatment is a basic understanding of the way drugs move through the body. Other topics include dosage adjustment, drug interactions, tolerance, and side effects. Using the treatment of hyperactivity as an example, an argument is made for the importance of caregiver participation in drug therapy.

Chapter 2: Hyperactivity. The most common childhood disorder for which psychotropic drugs are prescribed is hyperactivity. *Hyperactivity* is defined as a persistent developmental pattern characterized by excessive motor restlessness and inattentiveness. The latter may be the most important feature of the disorder. Other behavioral symptoms are frequently associated with hyperactivity, including poor school achievement, conduct problems, immaturity, impulsivity, and peer difficulties. In this chapter, research investigating the effects of stimulants (Ritalin, Dexedrine, and Cylert) on activity level, perceptual-motor skills, learning and cognitive performance, conduct problems, school achievement, and interpersonal relationships is summarized. The results of long-term followup studies on hyperactive children are also reviewed. Nonstimulant drugs occasionally used in the treatment of hyperactivity and nondrug therapies are also described briefly.

Chapter 3: Learning Disabilities. On the basis of available prevalence data, there are more children receiving special education services for learning disabilities in the United States than any other handicapping condition. The disorder is defined as a significant discrepancy between ability and academic achievement. Although there are no drugs specifically approved for the treatment of learning disabilities as defined by federal law, much has been written about the effects of stimulant drugs on academic performance in hyperactive children. This chapter discusses the relevant literature on this topic and the limited research on medication for nonhyperactive learning disabled children.

Chapter 4: Mental Retardation. Drug treatment for behavior disorders is much more common among mentally retarded children and adolescents in comparison with their nonretarded peers. Surveys show that stimulants are the most commonly prescribed drugs for behavior disorders in mentally retarded children in public school programs, whereas neuroleptics are the preferred agents in residential facilities. Some of the commonly reported reasons for administering medication are the control of hyperactivity, aggressivity, self-injurious behavior, and stereotypies. This chapter describes the use of neuroleptics (e.g., Thorazine, Mellaril, and Haldol) and stimulants in the treatment of behavior disorders associated with mental retardation. Many of the issues concerning the use of psychotropic drugs with mentally retarded people are discussed, including recent litigation.

Chapter 5: Early Childhood. Prescribing psychotropic drugs for children under 6 years of age is associated with a greater degree of uncertainty because little formal research is conducted with this age group for a number of obvious reasons. In spite of this situation, many preschool-aged children receive psychotropic medication, the two major categories being stimulants and neuroleptics. In this chapter the available literature on medication use with young children is reviewed to include existing treatment practices, clinical research, and the special issues that pertain to this population.

REFERENCES

Bradley, C. (1957). Characteristics and management of children with behavior problems associated with organic brain damage. *Pediatric Clinics of North America, 4,* 1049–1060.

Campbell, M., Anderson, L. T., & Green, W. H. (1983). Behavior-disordered and aggressive children: New advances in pharmacotherapy. *Developmental and Behavioral Pediatrics, 4,* 265–271.

Durack, D. T. (1978). The weight of medical knowledge. *New England Journal of Medicine, 298,* 773–775.

Epstein, M. H., Cullinan, D., & Gadow, K. D. (1985). *Prevalence of psychotropic drug use with learning disabled, emotionally disturbed, and mentally retarded children.* Unpublished manuscript, University of Northern Illinois, Department of Learning, Development, & Special Education, De Kalb.

Gadow, K. D. (1981). Prevalence of drug treatment for hyperactivity and other childhood behavior disorders. In K. D. Gadow & J. Loney (Eds.), *Psychosocial aspects of drug treatment for hyperactivity* (pp. 13–76). Boulder, CO: Westview Press.

Gadow, K. D. (1982a). Problems with students on medication. *Exceptional Children, 49,* 20–27.

Gadow, K. D. (1982b). School involvement in the treatment of seizure disorders. *Epilepsia, 23,* 215–224.

Gualtieri, C. T., Golden, R. N., & Fahs, J. J. (1983). New developments in pediatric psychopharmacology. *Developmental and Behavioral Pediatrics, 4,* 202–209.

Safer, D. J., & Krager, J. M. (1984). Trends in medication therapy for hyperactivity: National and international perspectives. In K. D. Gadow (Ed.), *Advances in learning and behavioral disabilities* (Vol. 3, pp. 125–149). Greenwich, CT: JAI Press.

Silverman, M., & Lee, P. R. (1974). *Pills, profits, and politics.* Berkeley: University of California Press.

Sprague, R. L., & Gadow, K. D. (1976). The role of the teacher in drug treatment. *School Review, 85,* 109–140.

Chapter 1

Fundamental Concepts in Pharmacotherapy: An Overview

There are approximately 10,000 prescription drugs available to American physicians, and an additional 100,000 products can be purchased without a prescription (Silverman & Lee, 1974). The latter are referred to as *over-the-counter* drugs or more simply as OTCs. Of the prescription medicines, two categories are of particular interest because they have pronounced effects upon behavior and are used frequently in treating chronic childhood disorders. These are the *psychotropic* and *antiepileptic* drugs.

Drugs that are prescribed primarily for their effect on mood, thought processes, and behavior are collectively referred to as psychotropic drugs. They include the *stimulants*, *neuroleptics* (major tranquilizers), *antianxiety agents* (minor tranquilizers), *antidepressants*, *hypnotics*, and *sedatives*. An extensive listing of the drugs in each of these categories appears in Appendix A. A seventh category of psychotropic agents, the *hallucinogens*, have not proved effective in the treatment of childhood disorders.

Antiepileptic drugs are used in the management of seizure disorders, and they can be further subdivided according to similarities in chemical structure. Because many psychotropic drugs have antiepileptic properties, there is considerable overlap between these two groups. To simplify matters, drugs used primarily for seizure disorders will be referred to as antiepileptics and the rest will be referred to as psychotropics. It would be inappropriate, however, to infer the reason for which a drug is prescribed from its assigned categorical label. For example, the antidepressant Tofranil (imipramine) is used

1

not only in the management of depression but also to treat spontaneous panic attacks (Klein et al., 1980), enuresis (Blackwell & Currah, 1973), hyperactivity (Rapoport et al., 1974), separation anxiety (Gittelman-Klein, 1975), and even certain types of seizure disorders (Fromm et al., 1978).

To add to the confusion, drugs have both a *generic* name and a *trade* name. As was noted in the Introduction, the generic name is typically used in the medical literature and is employed by the scientific community throughout the world. The trade name, however, is a registered trademark and is controlled by the manufacturer indefinitely. For reasons already discussed, drugs are referred to here by their United States trade name. In the case of drugs that are no longer protected by a patent, the original trade name is cited. After the first mention of a drug in each chapter, the generic name appears in parentheses.

Because generic products are often sold at a lower price than the original trade name product, compelling arguments have been made for more widespread use of generic drugs (Burack & Fox, 1975). In many states, the pharmacist can fill a doctor's prescription with a less expensive generic product unless the physician specifies no substitutions (Sonnenreich & Menger, 1977). (The actual guidelines for making substitutions vary from state to state.) The patient, of course, can always ask the doctor to write the prescription using the generic name if generic products are available. For this and other reasons, an extensive list of psychotropic and antiepileptic drugs by trade name appears in Appendix D along with the corresponding generic name.

CLASSIFICATION OF PSYCHOTROPIC DRUGS

Stimulants are among the most frequently prescribed psychotropic drugs for children and are used primarily for the management of hyperactivity. This group includes Ritalin (methylphenidate), Dexedrine (dextroamphetamine), and Cylert (pemoline). These drugs are occasionally used in the treatment of certain types of epilepsy and may be administered to control drowsiness, which is a side effect of some antiepileptic drugs. Stimulants are also used to treat *narcolepsy*, a disorder characterized by sudden attacks of sleep during normal waking hours. However, narcolepsy is an uncommon disorder and rarely develops in children under 12 years of age.

Neuroleptics are typically administered to control bizarre behavior in psychotic adults. These drugs are also referred to as *major tranquilizers* and *antipsychotic* agents. There are over a dozen neuroleptics that are used with some frequency, but the most common are Mellaril (thioridazine), Thorazine (chlorpromazine), and Haldol (haloperidol). In children, these drugs are administered to control hyperactivity, aggressivity, self-injurious behavior, and stereotypies and to facilitate in general management. Compared with children in regular classrooms, surveys show that neuroleptics are used more frequently to control behavior disorders in mentally retarded and emotionally disturbed children in special education programs.

Antianxiety agents (also called *minor tranquilizers* or *sedative-antianxiety* agents) can be subdivided into three major groups of drugs that share similar properties. One category is the *benzodiazepines* which includes Valium (diazepam), Librium (chlordiazepoxide), Clonopin (clonazepam), Serax (oxazepam), and Tranxene (clorazepate). All have antiepileptic properties, but Valium (one of the most frequently used prescription drugs in the world) and Clonopin are more commonly used with epileptic children. Valium is also a frequently prescribed skeletal muscle relaxant for children with cerebral palsy. At relatively high doses, Valium has hypnotic properties and, therefore, may be administered to induce sleep. *Diphenylmethane derivatives*, a second category of antianxiety agents, includes Atarax (hydroxyzine hydrochloride) and Vistaril (hydroxyzine pamoate). They are infrequently used to control hyperactivity, and, in younger children, they may be administered to induce sleep. A third category, *propanediols*, includes Equanil (meprobamate) and related drugs. Although they are frequently prescribed for anxiety in adults, surveys show they are not used very often with children. The benzodiazepines are preferred over the propanediols for the treatment of anxiety because the latter are more apt to be fatal in suicide attempts and accidental poisonings.

Among the antidepressant drugs, there are two major categories, one of which, the *tricyclics*, is relevant to this discussion. As previously stated, the term *antidepressant* is somewhat misleading, considering the variety of disorders for which these drugs are used. In children, Tofranil is the most frequently prescribed tricyclic drug. It is prescribed most often in the treatment of enuresis and occasionally for hyperactivity. Elavil (amitriptyline) is another tricyclic that may be used for hyperactivity but is more commonly prescribed for the treatment of depression in adolescents and adults. The other category of antidepressant drugs is the *monoamine oxidase inhibitors*, usually abbreviated MAOIs. They are used primarily with adults, typically for the treatment of depression.

Sedative drugs are used to calm anxious people and hypnotics are prescribed to induce sleep. The separation of these two categories is somewhat artificial because higher doses of most sedative drugs (e.g., antianxiety agents) have hypnotic effects. One large group of hypnotic drugs, the barbiturates, has antiepileptic properties. In fact, phenobarbital and Mebaral (mephobarbital) are used in children primarily to treat epilepsy. Examples of nonbarbiturate hypnotics are Noctec (chloral hydrate), Paral (paraldehyde), and Doriden (glutethimide).

Effective pharmacotherapy for seizure and behavior disorders is a fairly recent development. In the case of seizure disorders, it was not until the discovery of the antiepileptic properties of phenobarbital (Hauptmann, 1912) and Dilantin (Merritt & Putnam, 1938) that truly safe and powerful treatments were available. The first report of a highly effective agent specifically for the treatment of absence (petit mal) seizures was not published until World War II (Lennox, 1945). As for behavior and psychiatric disorders, the picture is similar. Prior to the discoveries that stimulants (Bradley, 1937) and neuroleptics (Heuyer et al., 1953) were powerful therapeutic agents for children, clinicians generally had to rely on sedatives, which often produced marked drowsiness and left the patient in a state of mental dullness or confusion.

PHARMACOKINETICS: MOVEMENT OF DRUGS IN THE BODY

In order for a drug to exert its characteristic effect, it must be absorbed into the body and transported to the tissues and organs in which it typically concentrates. For the effect to be terminated, the drug must be changed into an inactive substance or removed from the body. The movement of drugs into, through, and out of the body can be described in terms of four processes: *absorption* (movement into the blood), *distribution* (concentration in body compartments), *biotransformation* (breakdown of drugs into compounds that can be more readily removed), and *excretion* (movement out of the body).

Drugs can be administered either by mouth (orally) or by injection (*parenterally*). The latter method includes injecting the drug through various routes, such as *intravenously* (into the bloodstream); *subcutaneously* (under the surface of the skin); and *intramuscularly* (into muscle tissue). Intravenous injections can produce relatively immediate effects because the process of absorption in the gastrointestinal tract is bypassed. When injected into a muscle, drugs are absorbed into the bloodstream via the capillaries in the muscle tissue. The rate of absorption can be increased by adding a substance that dilates blood vessels or decreased with an agent that constricts them. Occasionally, neuroleptics are administered intramuscularly in a form that is not very soluble. This slows the rate of absorption, which in turn prolongs the effects of a single injection for several days. Subcutaneous injections are not used very often in the treatment of childhood medical disorders.

Absorption

Psychotropic and antiepileptic drugs are usually taken orally. This is the oldest and easiest route of drug administration. To be absorbed, drugs in tablet or capsule form must dissolve in the fluids of the stomach and intestine. Drug molecules then pass through the cells that line the wall of the digestive tract and into the capillaries of the veins that lead from the stomach to the liver.

A number of variables influence the rate of absorption, including the chemical characteristics of the drug, changes in the acidity of the stomach, other drugs present in the digestive tract, less than adequate supply of blood, and illnesses that result in a more rapid passage of food through the gut. Natural and added chemicals in the food we eat may also slow down or speed up this process. Because it is difficult to predict exactly how any change in the stomach or intestine may affect absorption, it is best to avoid, when possible, anything that might interfere with this process. For this reason, some drugs are administered at least 1 hour before or 2 hours after eating.

Distribution

Once in the bloodstream, drug molecules are distributed throughout the body, concentrating in various areas referred to as *compartments*. The characteristics of the drug determine the sites of distribution and the degree of concentration. Some agents are restricted primarily to the circulatory system. Others pass through the capillary membrane into the water that surrounds the tissues and cells (the extracellular fluid) or concentrate in the water inside the cells (intracellular fluid) of specific types of tissue.

The molecules of most drugs combine with large molecules in the blood (plasma protein). This process is referred to as *plasma protein binding*. Bound molecules, because of their size, are unable to pass out of the bloodstream, and, unlike unbound (free) drug molecules, do not have a pharmacological effect on the body. An equilibrium is established between bound and unbound molecules. As free molecules pass out of the blood, bound molecules are released so that the ratio of bound to unbound molecules in the blood remains the same. Although the maximal effect of the drug is reduced by protein binding, it prolongs the effect of the drug by creating a reservoir of bound drug molecules that are released over time (Briant, 1978).

The movement of drug molecules from the bloodstream into the brain is made more difficult by the presence of a *blood-brain barrier.* This is not an anatomical structure per se but refers to the fact that the capillaries of the brain prevent certain classes of compounds from entering and affecting brain neurones. A closeknit layer of glial cells surrounds the brain capillaries, creating an additional barrier for compounds that are not lipid soluble. Without such a barrier, many chemicals in the foods we eat could directly alter the function of the central nervous system. Examples of agents that do pass through the blood-brain barrier are psychotropic and antiepileptic drugs.

Biotransformation

The liver is the primary organ responsible for the breakdown of drugs (biotransformation) into new compounds (metabolites). Substances (*microsomal enzymes*) within the cells of the liver bring about or increase the rate of the chemical reactions that transform drugs into metabolites. Generally, an active drug is metabolized into an inactive, more water soluble compound that can be excreted through the kidney. If lipid soluble drugs (e.g., Valium) were not transformed into water-soluble metabolites, they would be reabsorbed into the bloodstream by the kidney, and the effects of a single dose could, therefore, last indefinitely (Briant, 1978).

Not all drugs are metabolized into inactive substances within the body. Some are excreted unchanged, whereas others are transformed from inert substances into active metabolites. An example of the latter is the antiepileptic drug Mysoline (primidone), which does not appear to be effective in the treatment of epilepsy in its initial form (Callaghan et al., 1977). However, drug-metabolizing enzymes in the liver convert Mysoline into active metabolites, which in turn control seizures.

The rate of drug metabolism in the liver can be greatly affected by the presence of another drug or chemical. This is one form of drug interaction. Genetic factors also play an important role in determining the speed at which compounds are transformed. When the same drug is administered to a number of different people, the rate of metabolism may vary greatly (Vessell & Page, 1968).

Excretion

The kidney is the primary organ responsible for the removal of drugs and their metabolites from the body in the form of water-soluble compounds. Other pathways of elimination are feces, perspiration, and the milk of nursing mothers.

The rate of excretion can be influenced by the pH of the urine. For example, basic drug molecules are excreted more rapidly when the urine is acidic, and vice versa. Therefore, the presence of another drug or chemical that changes the pH of the urine could alter the rate of excretion.

Many, but certainly not all, drugs have *linear kinetics*, which means that the body's drug elimination mechanisms excrete a constant amount or percentage of the drug per unit of time. One of the most widely used expressions to describe drug elimination is *half-life*, which is the amount of time it takes the body to reduce the amount of drug in the blood by 50%. For drugs with linear kinetics, the half-life is *independent* of both dose and concentration. The average half-life is a useful guide for therapy because it takes five half-lives to reach a stable concentration *(steady state)* of drug in the blood after treatment has been initiated (see, for example, Table 2–5). A steady state is attained when the rate of drug intake is equal to the rate of output (removal from the body). Although blood concentrations do fluctuate between doses, during a steady state they are fairly stable. This is most important because a particular medication generally cannot be adequately evaluated until a stable drug concentration has been reached. Knowing the half-life is also useful when medication is withdrawn because it takes approximately five half-lives for a drug to be completely eliminated from the body. It is also a helpful guide for dosing. When a drug is administered once per half-life, this will generally prevent wide fluctuations in drug blood concentrations.

Some drugs have *nonlinear kinetics*, which means their elimination mechanisms can become saturated. In other words, as the dose or concentration of the drug increases, the body eliminates more drug, only at a slower rate. Therefore, the apparent half-life increases. This complicates the picture because for any age group there is a wide range of half-lives depending upon the dose and the initial concentration at which the apparent half-life is measured. An excellent example of a commonly prescribed antiepileptic drug that has nonlinear kinetics is Dilantin (phenytoin). For more discussion on how information about drug kinetics and blood concentrations are used in making clinical decisions, see Dodson (1984) and Gualtieri et al. (1984).

DOSAGE

Before a drug is marketed, a considerable amount of information is collected about the effects of different amounts of the drug on laboratory animals and people. From reports of accidental poisonings and suicide attempts, it is even possible to determine fatal human dosage levels. In adjusting dosage, the physician starts with a small amount of the medication—usually below the therapeutic range. Over time, the dose is gradually increased until the desired response is achieved. This process is referred to as *titration*. Recommended dosage limits, both minimum and maximum, guide the physician in this procedure. If unwanted or intolerable side effects emerge, (a) the dose may have to be reduced; (b) the drug may be stopped completely and gradually reintroduced; (c) a different medication may be substituted for the offending agent; or (d) an additional drug may be prescribed to control the side effect.

People differ from one another internally as well as externally. Individual variability in the way we react to drugs may reflect differences in the biological systems that are responsible for absorption, distribution, biotransformation, and excretion or simply differences in body size. In order to limit some of this variability in drug response, researchers sometimes adjust dosage to physical size. A measured amount of medication is administered per unit of body weight in kilograms (kg). A kilogram equals approximately 2.2 pounds.

Medication is typically measured in milligrams (mg). One milligram is equivalent to approximately 1/28,000 of an ounce. The actual dosage in milligrams per kilogram of body weight (mg/kg) can be calculated as follows: $DW = M$, where D = desired mg/kg dose, W = weight in kilograms, and M = actual amount of medication in milligrams. For example, assume the physician decides to administer drug A at a dose of 0.3 mg/kg. A child weighing 88 pounds (40 kg) would then receive 12 mg of drug A ($DW = M$; 0.3 × 40 = 12). For any given M, the mg/kg dose can be determined by a simple algebraic manipulation. Thus, for a child who weighs 44 pounds (20 kg) and is receiving 12 mg of drug A each morning, the dose would be 0.6 mg/kg ($\frac{M}{W} = D$; 12/20 = 0.6).

With some drugs, particularly the antiepileptics, the amount of medication administered in milligrams has little relationship with the amount in the blood. For example, if a number of people with epilepsy are given the same dose of Dilantin, the actual level in the blood would vary greatly from patient to patient (Lascelles et al.,

1970). Therefore, a more useful measure than mg/kg for dose would be one that indicated how much drug was in the blood. That measure is the amount of drug, in micrograms (mcg or μg) for example, per milliliter (ml) of blood. These are very small amounts. For example, there are 1,000 micrograms in 1 milligram. An even smaller unit of measurement is the *nanogram*. There are 1,000 micrograms in 1 nanogram. When expressed as an amount in the blood, it is often cited as nanograms per milliliter (ng/ml).

Monitoring blood levels of antiepileptic drugs is an important procedure in the effective management of many children with epilepsy (Kutt, 1974). In contrast, psychotropic drug treatment is not typically monitored in this way (see Gualtieri et al., 1984). In fact, procedures for determining blood levels are not yet available for many of these agents. It is noteworthy that a reliable method for assessing blood levels of Ritalin in children is a fairly recent development.

SIDE EFFECTS

No drug is completely free of side effects. There are a number of terms used to denote side effects, including *untoward reactions, toxic effects,* and *adverse drug reactions.* There is also a newer term, *treatment emergent symptoms,* that is being popularized to some extent in the psychiatry literature. Some side effects are trivial, whereas others seriously impair health. The latter are sometimes referred to as *toxic effects,* but this term appears to be used somewhat inconsistently. Adverse effects may go away after a period of time (*self-limiting*) or they may persist. If the disorder being treated is severe, side effects that are not self-limiting may have to be endured. Side effects may appear shortly after the onset of treatment or may go unrecognized for months or even years. The pervasiveness of side effects often alarms people, but one must realize that the body is an extremely complicated chemical system whose functions are highly interrelated and that the alteration of one process affects others as well. It is noteworthy that what is an adverse drug reaction for one person may be the desired treatment response for another patient with a different disorder.

When drugs interfere with a person's ability to think, interact socially, and perform work-related behaviors (classroom activities in the case of children) or either induce or aggravate (*exacerbate*) a preexisting behavior disorder, this reaction is often referred to as *behavioral toxicity.* Unfortunately, such reactions often occur at dosages below or at therapeutic levels. In recent years, much deserved attention has been focused on behavioral toxicity with regard to *risk-to-benefit* decisions. In other words, do the benefits of drug therapy outweigh the risks? The latter consists of short-term side effects that are immediately evident as well as longer-term adverse reactions that are not apparent until long after the commitment to therapy has been made. Some long-term consequences of treatment are really the cumulative effects of chronic drug-induced impairment. Because the signs or symptoms of behavioral toxicity are often difficult to detect on the basis of behavior exhibited in the physician's office but may be clearly visible to the care providers, this topic has received special attention in this book.

Most side effects are predictable. They may take the form of (a) an excessive therapeutic response that can typically be corrected by dosage reduction or (b) physiological or behavioral reactions that are commonly associated with the pharmacological properties of the drug. For example, aggressive children treated with neuroleptic drugs may become abnormally inactive (excessive therapeutic response) or may experience a temporary dryness of the mouth due to the drug's characteristic effect on the autonomic nervous system (pharmacologically predictable response). Other, less common side effects are not predictable because they are due, in part, to the genetic or physiological peculiarities of the patient (*host factor*). One such side effect is an *allergic* reaction also called *hypersensitivity*. Skin reactions are a common sign of drug allergy. Another unpredictable side effect is an *idiosyncratic* reaction, which is characterized by an excessive or abnormal unexplained response to a typical dose of medication.

DOSE-RESPONSE

As we all know from our experiences with either common substances such as coffee and alcoholic beverages or with prescription and nonprescription medication, the amount of drug intake is directly related to the experienced effect. Whereas one cup of coffee may make us more alert for our drive to work, several cups during a short period may leave us nervous and overly responsive to mild stress. This relationship between dose and drug effect is referred to as *dose-response* or *dose-effect*. Although this may sound fairly straightforward, it is not. The complicating variable is that drugs almost always produce multiple physiological and behavioral effects. Moreover, the dose-response *and* time-course relationships for these various treatment effects often differ.

This concept can be better appreciated by examining Figure 1–1, which is an adaptation of hypothetical dose-response relations for stimulant drugs in hyperactive children proposed by Sprague and Sleator (1975). They are presented here as more general response patterns to portray treatment issues associated with most psychotropic and antiepileptic drugs. The target symptom curve represents any of the behavioral features for which these drugs are prescribed (e.g., seizures, aggressivity, school phobia, activity level). As the dosage increases, symptom control becomes greater and greater. There reaches a point, however, after which further dosage increments fail to improve the condition, at least to any appreciable degree. Equally important is that there is an optimal range of dosages that produce a fairly similar degree of therapeutic improvement. For example, if the optimal range is 150 to 200 mg, the amount of improvement obtained with the larger dose is fairly similar to that for the lower dose. This idea of an optimal range has caused some people to argue that it makes more sense to use a *smaller* dose from the optimal range, particularly when side effects are an issue.

The descending part of the target symptom curve is shown as a dashed line because higher drug dosages may or may not exacerbate the target symptoms. For example, higher therapeutic dosages of Dilantin may actually cause an *increase* in seizure frequency (Levy & Fenichel, 1965), which would be represented as a decrease in improvement or a descending slope. For many other target symptoms, however, higher therapeutic dosages generally do not lead to a deterioration (e.g., increased frequency) in the symptoms for which the drug was prescribed. Unfortunately, the same cannot be said for adaptive behavior.

Because the ability to think clearly, solve problems, learn, and interact socially is so important to everyday life, drug-induced impairment of these behaviors are considered to be a serious treatment-related consideration. It goes without saying that this is particularly true for children in general and for people with limited intellectual ability. The adaptive behavior curve in Figure 1–1 depicts two possible outcomes. One, the drug may actually enhance adaptive behavior even though this may *not* be the primary target of intervention (dotted line). Such outcomes should be considered *serendipitous* (accidental but nevertheless beneficial) but often have a way of becoming justifications for treatment. As is evident from the figure, medication enhances adaptive behavior, but with increasing dosage all the beneficial effects are nullified and performance drops even below baseline levels (dashed line) at higher dosages.

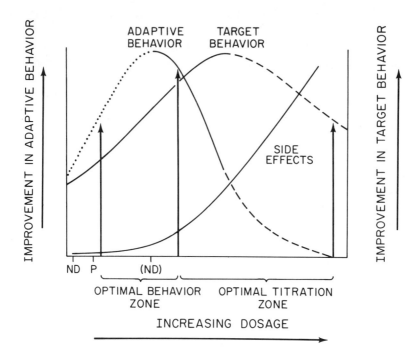

Figure 1-1. Dose-response relationships for target symptoms, adaptive behavior, and somatic side effects for a hypothetical drug. From "What is the proper dose of stimulant drugs in children?" R. L. Sprague, & E. K. Sleator (1975). *International Journal of Mental Health, 4,* p. 96. Copyright 1975 by International Arts & Sciences Press, Inc. Adapted by permission.

Although this type of reaction is rarely reported for psychotropic drugs other than the stimulants (e.g., Sprague & Sleator, 1977), it has been found with neuroleptic drugs as well (e.g., Werry & Aman, 1975) and certainly depends, in part, on task characteristics. As with target symptoms, there is an optimal dosage range. Ideally, therapeutic gain is maximized by selection of a dosage that benefits both adaptive and target behaviors.

Probably the more typical situation with adaptive behaviors is represented by the solid adaptive behavior line and the second baseline, which is designated in Figure 1-1 as (ND). In this case, the therapist does not anticipate improvement in adaptive behavior but is concerned about the extent to which adaptive behavior is *impaired* by medication (i.e., behavioral toxicity). In our example, only mild impairment is seen at the lower end of the therapeutic dosage range for treating target symptoms.

The side effects line in this figure represents somatic symptoms (e.g., heart rate, dizziness, double vision, and so forth). It is placed to the right of the behavioral toxicity curve because it has been hypothesized (e.g., Sprague & Werry, 1971) that behavioral toxicity may be more commonly manifested at dosages lower than those associated with serious somatic complaints. It should be evident from this example that dosage titration on the basis of somatic side effects could lead to medication levels that severely impair adaptive behavior. Although this may sound fairly simple, in real-world situations it is often very difficult to effectively evaluate behavioral toxicity, therapeutic response, and in some instances, even somatic toxicity.

TOLERANCE

When the same dose of medication no longer has a characteristic effect after repeated administrations, this is referred to as *tolerance*. Because drugs often have many properties, children may develop a tolerance for only some of them. For example, although children typically develop a tolerance for the drowsiness produced by phenobarbital, the seizure-controlling properties of the drug may not change. Although adjustments are typically made in the dosage of antiepileptic drugs as the child grows to accommodate to changes in body size, this is not the same thing as tolerance.

Repeated drug administrations may also increase the rate at which drugs move through the body. This is referred to as *drug disposition* or *metabolic tolerance*. For example, the regular intake of some drugs actually stimulates the metabolic processes responsible for the breakdown of the drug. To achieve the same effect, the dose must be larger than the previous one. This may only increase the rate of biotransformation and the cycle is repeated. In one study of epileptic adults treated with Dilantin, 45% showed a drop in the blood level of the drug over several months of treatment (Reynolds et al., 1976). In some cases, the level dropped so low that seizures recurred in patients who were previously seizure free. The situation was remedied by increasing the dose. It should be noted, however, that in the treatment of epilepsy, this does *not* typically end in a vicious cycle of dosage increments.

Pharmacodynamic or *cellular tolerance* develops when the cells of the nervous system actually adjust to the presence of the medication. In order to achieve the same reaction to the drug, the dosage must be increased to overcome the body's compensatory mechanisms. If a neurological adjustment is made to the larger dose, even more medication will be required, and so forth. This type of tolerance is encountered with the euphoric effect of opium and related drugs.

DEPENDENCE AND ADDICTION

Another reaction associated with the repeated use of certain drugs is *physical dependence*. This occurs when an agent alters the physiological state of the body, and, to prevent the appearance of a *withdrawal syndrome*, the drug must continue to be administered. Physical dependence has been demonstrated with a number of drugs including opiates, barbiturates, alcohol, amphetamines, and nicotine (Jaffe, 1980). Because the symptoms that characterize the withdrawal syndrome are associated with the same area of the body that was initially altered by the drug and are often the complete opposite of the drug effect, they are sometimes referred to as *rebound effects*. For example, the sudden cessation of an antiepileptic drug (e.g., phenobarbital) may precipitate a seizure. This can be avoided by simply lowering the dose of medication over an extended period of time before stopping treatment.

The difference between physical dependence and *drug addiction* is not often made clear. Drug addiction refers to a "behavioral pattern of drug use, characterized by overwhelming involvement with the use of a drug (compulsive use), the securing of its supply, and a high tendency to relapse after withdrawal" (Jaffe, 1980, p. 536). It is important to note that a person can be physically dependent upon a drug and *not* be addicted, or be addicted and *not* be physically dependent.

Parents and teachers often worry whether children receiving psychotropic or antiepileptic medication are addicted. They are not! Nor are they more apt to become drug users in later life.

DRUG INTERACTIONS

It is not unusual for children to receive two or more different drugs during the same day. Some disorders may require more than one medicine to achieve a satisfactory therapeutic response. For example, surveys of epileptic children in special education programs report that approximately half of the students receive two or more antiepileptic drugs per day (Gadow, 1982). Children may also have more than one disorder that requires long-term drug treatment. Studies show that from 7 to 10% of the children on medication in

special education programs receive drugs for both behavior and seizure disorders (Gadow, 1977; Gadow & Kalachnik, 1981). There are
also tens of thousands of nonprescription products available to parents for the treatment of common childhood maladies such as colds,
headaches, upset stomachs, and so forth. Although these products
are not always regarded as "drugs," the concomitant administration
of a prescription and a nonprescription medicine is a drug combination. Another situation for which a combination of drugs is used is
the management of unwanted drug reactions. For example, if a medicine causes serious side effects but cannot be stopped for therapeutic reasons, the physician may prescribe an additional drug
specifically to control the side effects.

The use of two different drugs for the same disorder, probably
best referred to as *multiple-drug therapy*, is generally unwarranted
and ill-advised unless (a) the two agents possess a different
mechanism of action and (b) the clinical utility of the two in
combination is clearly superior to either when used singly. Some
classic examples of effective multiple-drug therapy based on
independent mechanisms of action can be found in antimicrobial
therapy (see Sande & Mandell, 1980). Trimethoprim and
sulfamethoxazole are used in combination to treat lower urinary
tract infections because the two drugs interact *synergistically* (the
combination effect is greater than the sum effect of each drug when
used individually). Each interferes with a *different* step in the
production of folic acid in certain bacteria. Because there are few
truly compelling examples of useful multiple-drug therapy for
seizure or behavior disorders, this practice is generally frowned
upon.

Multiple drug use that arises out of the concurrent management
of two or more disorders (or symptoms) has also generated international concern. Reports of multiple drug use in residential facilities,
hospitals, and community care centers for the elderly or the mentally retarded have led some clinicians to question the necessity for
all of the drugs that are prescribed. Drug combinations in these settings are an important clinical consideration in that the effects of
one agent may be significantly altered by the presence of another.
When this does occur, it is referred to as drug *interaction*.

One way in which drugs interact is an alteration in the absorption, distribution, biotransformation, or excretion of one agent by
another (*pharmacokinetic interactions*). Changes in the rate at
which these processes occur can result in an increase or decrease in
the blood level of the altered drug. Several examples of drug interactions are presented here to better explain these processes.

If drug A slows down the rate at which drug B is absorbed into the blood, it will take longer for drug B to reach an effective level. This could be very important if it is necessary to obtain a high level of drug B in the bloodstream to be really effective for medical treatment. One example of this type of interaction is between milk or milk products and the antibiotic drug tetracycline. It is generally recommended that orally administered tetracycline be taken 1 hour before or 2 hours after meals because these foods can impair the absorption of tetracycline.

Once drug molecules have entered the bloodstream, another type of drug interaction becomes possible, and this involves plasma protein binding. If drug A is associated with a clinically significant degree of plasma protein binding, the addition of drug B to the treatment regimen could create problems if it also binds to plasma proteins and has greater affinity for the binding site than drug A. This situation could lead to a marked increase in the number of unbound (free) drug A molecules in the blood, which in turn could result in a rapid and dramatic increase in drug A effects (both therapeutic and adverse). Ironically, this heightened effect is typically short-lived because the free drug molecules are now also available for biotransformation or excretion (glomerular filtration) and the end result may be lower blood levels of drug A.

The rate at which drugs are broken down by the liver can also be altered. Many drugs, for example, inhibit the biotransformation of Dilantin (Kutt, 1972). Because Dilantin is poorly soluble in water, drug molecules must be transformed into water-soluble metabolites before they can be excreted by the kidney. Therefore, a drug that inhibits the metabolism of Dilantin produces an increase in the blood level of the latter. Because there are now more Dilantin molecules in general circulation, the effect is greater. This could result in unwanted side effects, fewer seizures if attacks were not completely controlled when Dilantin was administered alone, or both. When one drug inhibits the biotransformation of another, the consequences of this interaction are typically experienced within hours or days after the addition of the offending medication.

In addition to being inhibited, biotransformation can also be made to occur more rapidly (induced). One way this can happen is for one drug (B) to cause an increase in the production of the microsomal enzymes that break down another drug (A). When drug B is added to the treatment regimen, the blood level of drug A may drop because it is being converted into metabolites for excretion at a faster rate. This is generally a more gradual process and may not become clinically significant until after weeks or months of concurrent drug use.

Another type of drug interaction occurs when two drugs with similar effects are given in combination. For example, alcohol and barbiturates both produce central nervous system depression ranging from mild sedation to coma, depending on the amount consumed. When they are both used during the same period of time, their effects are *additive* and the outcome may be fatal. The combination of the two substances is similar to a much larger amount of either one ingested alone.

SUGGESTED READINGS

Abel, E. L. (1974). *Drugs and behavior: A primer in neuropsychopharmacology.* New York: Wiley. (C)

Campbell, M., Anderson, L. T., & Green, W. H. (1983). Behavior-disordered and aggressive children: New advances in pharmacotherapy. *Developmental and Behavioral Pediatrics, 4,* 265–271. (C, S)

Eisenberg, L. (1975). The ethics of intervention: Acting amidst ambiguity. *Journal of Child Psychology and Psychiatry, 16,* 93–104. (C)

Engel, G. L. (1977). The need for a new medical model: A challenge for biomedicine. *Science, 196,* 129–135. (C)

Gilman, A. G., Goodman, L. S., & Gilman, A. (Eds.). (1980). *The pharmacological basis of therapeutics* (6th ed.). New York: Macmillan. (C, S)

Gualtieri, C. T., Golden, R. N., & Fahs, J. J. (1983). New developments in pediatric psychopharmacology. *Developmental and Behavioral Pediatrics, 4,* 202–209. (C, S)

Klein, D. F., Gittelman, R., Quitkin, F., & Rifkin, A. (1980). *Diagnosis and drug treatment of psychiatric disorders: Adults and children* (2nd ed.). Baltimore: Williams & Wilkins. (C)

Leavitt, F. (1982). *Drugs and behavior* (2nd ed.). Philadelphia: Saunders. (C, S)

Silverman, M., & Lee, P. R. (1974). *Pills, profits, and politics.* Berkeley: University of California Press. (C, S)

Sprague, R. L., & Gadow, K. D. (1976). The role of the teacher in drug treatment. *School Review, 85,* 109–140. (S)

Werry, J. S. (Ed.). (1978). *Pediatric psychopharmacology: The use of behavior modifying drugs in children.* New York: Brunner/Mazel. (C)

REFERENCES

Blackwell, B., & Currah, J. (1973). The psychopharmacology of nocturnal enuresis. In I. Kolvin, R. C. MacKeith, & S. R. Meadow (Eds.), *Bladder control and enuresis* (pp. 231–257). Philadelphia: Lippincott.

Bradley, C. (1937). The behavior of children receiving Benzedrine. *American Journal of Psychiatry, 94,* 577–585.

Briant, R. H. (1978). An introduction to clinical pharmacology. In J. S. Werry (Ed.), *Pediatric psychopharmacology: The use of behavior modifying drugs in children* (pp. 3–28). New York: Brunner/Mazel.

Burack, R. B., & Fox, F. J. (1975). *The new handbook of prescription drugs* (rev. ed.). New York: Ballantine Books.

Callaghan, N., Feely, M., Duggan, F., O'Callaghan, M., & Seldrup, S. (1977). The effect of anticonvulsant drugs which induce liver microsomal enzymes on derived and ingested phenobarbitone levels. *Acta Neurologica Scandinavica, 56,* 1–6.

Dodson, W. E. (1984). Antiepileptic drug utilization in pediatric patients. *Epilepsia, 25* (Suppl. 2), S132–S139.

Fromm, G. H., Wessel, H. B., Glass, J. D., Alvin, J. D., & van Horn, G. (1978). Imipramine in absence and myoclonic-astatic seizures. *Neurology, 28,* 953–957.

Gadow, K. D. (1977). *Psychotropic and antiepileptic drug treatment with children in early childhood special education.* Champaign, IL: Institute for Child Behavior and Development, University of Illinois (ERIC Document Reproduction Service No. ED 162 294).

Gadow, K. D. (1982). School involvement in the treatment of seizure disorders. *Epilepsia, 23,* 215–224.

Gadow, K. D., & Kalachnik, J. (1981). Prevalence and pattern of drug treatment for behavior and seizure disorders of TMR students. *American Journal of Mental Deficiency, 85,* 588–595.

Gittelman-Klein, R. (1975). Pharmacotherapy and management of pathological separation anxiety. *International Journal of Mental Health, 4,* 255–271.

Gualtieri, C. T., Golden, R., Evans, R. W., & Hicks, R. E. (1984). Blood level measurement of psychoactive drugs in pediatric psychiatry. *Therapeutic Drug Monitoring, 6,* 127–141.

Hauptmann, A. (1912) Luminal boi Epilopsic. München. Med. Wschr., 59, 1907–1909.

Heuyer, G., Gerard, G., & Galibert, J. (1953). Traitement de l'excitation psychometrics chez l'enfant pare (le 4560 r.p.). *Archives Francaises de Pediatrie, 9,* 961.

Jaffe, J. H. (1980). Drug addiction and drug abuse. In A. G. Gilman, S. Goodman, & A. Gilman (Eds.), *The pharmacological basis of therapeutics* (6th ed.). New York: Macmillan.

Klein, D. F., Gittelman, R., Quitkin, F., & Rifkin, A. (1980). *Diagnosis and drug treatment of psychiatric disorders: Adults and children* (2nd ed.). Baltimore: Williams & Wilkins.

Kutt, H. (1972). Diphenylhydantoin: Interactions with other drugs in man. In D. M. Woodbury, J. K. Penry, & R. P. Schmidt (Eds.), *Antiepileptic drugs* (pp. 169–180). New York: Raven.

Kutt, H. (1974). The use of blood levels of antiepileptic drugs in clinical practice. *Pediatrics, 53,* 557–560.

Lascelles, P. T., Kocen, R. S., & Reynolds, E. H. (1970). The distribution of plasma phenytoin levels in epileptic patients. *Journal of Neurology, Neurosurgery and Psychiatry, 33,* 501–505.

Lennox, W. G. (1945). Treatment of epilepsy. *Medical Clinics of North America, 29,* 1114–1128.

Levy, L. L., & Fenichel, G. M. (1965). Diphenylhydantoin activated seizures. *Neurology, 15,* 716–722.

Merritt, H. H., & Putnam, T. J. (1938). Sodium diphenyl hydantoinate in the treatment of convulsive disorders. *Journal of the American Medical Association, 111*, 1068–1073.

Rapoport, J. L., Quinn, P. O., Bradbard, G., Riddle, K. D., & Brooks, E. (1974). Imipramine and methylphenidate treatments of hyperactive boys. *Archives of General Psychiatry, 30*, 789–793.

Reynolds, E. H., Chadwick, D., & Galbraith, A. W. (1976). One drug (phenytoin) in the treatment of epilepsy. *Lancet, 1*, 923–926.

Sande, M. A., & Mandell, G. L. (1980). Antimicrobial agents: General considerations. In A. G. Gilman, L. S. Goodman, & A. Gilman (Eds.), *The pharmacological basis of therapeutics* (6th ed., pp. 1080–1105). New York: Macmillan.

Silverman, M., & Lee, P. R. (1974). *Pills, profits, and politics.* Berkeley: University of California Press.

Sonnenreich, M. R., & Menger, J. M. (1977, April). State substitution laws: A lawyer's view. *U.S. Pharmacist*, pp. 18–23.

Sprague, R. L., & Sleator, E. K. (1975). What is the proper dose of stimulant drugs in children? *International Journal of Mental Health, 4*, 75–104.

Sprague, R. L., & Sleator, E. K. (1977). Methylphenidate in hyperkinetic children: Differences in dose effects on learning and social behavior. *Science, 198*, 1274–1276.

Sprague, R. L., & Werry, J. S. (1971). Methodology of psychopharmacological studies with the retarded. In N. R. Ellis (Ed.), *International review of research in mental retardation* (Vol. 5, pp. 147–219). Orlando, FL: Academic Press.

Vessell, E., & Page, J. (1968). Genetic control of drug levels in man: Antipyrine. *Science, 161*, 72–73.

Werry, J. S., & Aman, M. G. (1975). Methylphenidate and haloperidol in children. *Archives of General Psychiatry, 32*, 790–795.

Chapter **2**

Seizure Disorders

The primary symptom of a seizure disorder is, of course, a *seizure*. To an observer, a *seizure* is a sudden attack, usually manifested by a complete or partial loss of consciousness and accompanied by involuntary muscle movement or a cessation of body movement. If the seizure involves violent, involuntary contractions of skeletal muscles, it may be referred to as a convulsion. A distinction must therefore be made between convulsive (grand mal) and nonconvulsive (e.g., absence) seizures. The term *seizure*, however, refers to both.

Seizures are caused by a sudden discharge of electrical energy in the brain. The actual reason for these discharges and the great susceptibility to them for some people remains obscure. Anyone can have a seizure if the appropriate stimulus causes an electrical discharge in the brain. Examples of such stimuli are infections, poisons and drugs, sudden oxygen deprivation, and metabolic disturbances. Seizures are generally not considered to be symptoms of a seizure disorder unless they are recurring in nature. Recurring seizures are frequently referred to as *epilepsy*, and this is the preferred term for designating such seizures according to groups such as the Epilepsy Foundation of American and to many clinicians. However, it has been my experience that many parents use terms such as *seizures*, *convulsions*, and *spells* when referring to their child's disorder. In addition, these terms seem to be more behaviorally oriented in that they focus on the visible features of the disorder, the reason for which drugs are prescribed, and the yardstick against which the effectiveness of medication is measured (i.e., seizure suppression).

Recurrent seizures are sometimes classified according to what is known about their cause. If the cause of the seizures is unknown, they are said to be *idiopathic*. In approximately one fourth to one half of all cases of epilepsy, the cause of the seizures is unknown. Idiopathic epilepsy is more common among children with seizures, especially those over 4 years old, than among adults. Seizures that develop as a result of permanent, nonprogressive changes or damage to the brain are called *secondary* or *organic* epilepsy. For example, seizures that occurred subsequent to a head injury sustained in an automobile accident would be considered secondary. It should not be inferred that the head trauma is the sole cause of the disorder, because not all children with equal degrees of head injury develop seizures. It is quite possible there is a complex interaction between an unknown factor or factors and the trauma that leads to a seizure disorder. This same unknown entity may also cause idiopathic epilepsy.

The actual sensory and motor phenomena associated with a seizure depend upon which cells in the brain are affected by the abnormal electrical discharge. If the discharge is initially confined to one area in one hemisphere of the brain, the seizure is said to be *partial*. Symptoms of the attack might be the twitching of a finger or arm, a strange sensation, or a change in mood. If the electrical activity affects the entire brain, the resulting seizures are said to be generalized. Two examples of generalized seizures are tonic-clonic (grand mal) and absence (petit mal). It should be noted that a seizure could originate as a partial seizure but progress into a generalized seizure, in which case it is said to be *secondarily* generalized. For example, a true *Jacksonian* seizure, rarely found in children, is a partial seizure that may begin by a twitching in a finger of the right hand, which progresses to jerking movements of the hand and right arm, then to twitching movements on the right side of the face continuing on down the same side of the body (Livingston, 1972). During this part of the attack, the individual usually remains conscious. The seizure is partial in that specific motor areas of the brain are affected. These jerking or clonic movements may then spread to the opposite side of the body as the electrical discharge moves to the previously unaffected hemisphere of the brain. At this point, consciousness is lost. The electrical discharge may then spread throughout the brain, culminating in a generalized tonic-clonic seizure.

Much of the discussion in this chapter is based on the clinical experience and research efforts of Dr. Samuel Livingston. His publications provide not only a broad data base but also a consistent conceptualization of the field. Because there are a number of inconsistencies in the literature about seizure disorders and the variety of treatment techniques employed by physicians, Livingston's position is used as a standard against which other opinions are compared (Livingston, 1972, 1978a, 1978b).

PREVALENCE OF SEIZURE DISORDERS

For a number of reasons, there is considerable variability in the prevalence of seizure disorders reported from study to study. Actual prevalence rates range from 1.5 to 20 cases per 1,000, with a median of 3.8 people with epilepsy for every 1,000 in the general population (Meighan et al., 1976). However, many epileptologists believe most prevalence studies underestimate the true extent of seizure disorders. Livingston (1972), for example, estimated that 1 in 50 Americans have epilepsy at some time during their lives. Similarly, the Epilepsy Foundation of America (1975) has adopted a 2% prevalence rate for seizure disorders in the general population.

One of the reasons some studies may have underestimated the extent of this disorder is that untreated persons are frequently excluded from surveys and, of course, some cases go undiagnosed. More recently, efforts have been made to detect undiagnosed and untreated cases of epilepsy. Using a combination of diagnostic and survey techniques, Rose et al. (1973), for example, reported a "reasonable" prevalence rate of 18.6 cases of epilepsy per 1,000 among third grade children.

Although dozens of studies have been conducted on the prevalence of epilepsy per se, there are few published statements about the prevalence of drug treatment for this disorder among school-aged children. Assuming the prevalence figures based on school children identified and treated for seizure disorders are also a fairly accurate description of the extent of drug use, between 0.3 and 0.6% of the students in regular classrooms are on medication for epilepsy (Force, 1965). The figures for many types of special education programs are, however, much higher (see Chapter 3).

At least three-fourths of all the people with epilepsy experienced their first seizure before the age of 20 (Lennox, 1960). The highest incidence rates (number of new cases) are for infants from birth and 2 years, children between the ages of 5 and 7, and adolescents (the onset of puberty). The latter is particularly true for females who may experience seizures with their first menstruation (Livingston, 1972).

DIAGNOSIS

Although electroencephalographic (EEG) recordings are typically associated with the diagnosis of seizure disorders, in the majority of cases the most important diagnostic information is going to be caregiver descriptions of child behavior (Stores, 1985). This is true because children with seizure disorders rarely exhibit seizures in the physician's office or during an EEG recording session. The latter is problematical because the *interictal* (between seizures) EEG is often normal (e.g., Ajmone Marsan & Zivin, 1970). Nevertheless, the EEG pattern is *pathognomic* (a sign or symptom for making a diagnosis) for certain types of seizure disorders, is useful in monitoring response to treatment and changes in clinical course, and "is essential in the initial evaluation of seizure disorders" (Lee, 1983, p. 33). The EEG has special utility for the diagnosis of nonconvulsive seizures that take the form of behavioral or cognitive aberrations and for differentiating between hysterical or pseudoseizures from true seizures and nonepileptic disorders from true epileptic phenomena. The development of ambulatory monitoring systems (Stores, 1985) that the child can simply wear (electrodes hidden under hair; wires concealed under clothing, and recorder worn on belt) is creating a small revolution in the diagnosis of difficult cases. For a truly lucid and beautifully prepared discussion of the role of EEG monitoring in childhood epilepsy, the reader is referred to a chapter by Lee (1983).

CLASSIFICATION OF SEIZURE DISORDERS

Most seizure disorders can be categorized as belonging to one of several groups. There are, however, a number of different classification schemes, and often several different terms are used to denote the same seizure type. For lay people and professionals alike, this proliferation of terms creates both confusion and misunderstanding. This problem is not peculiar to the study of seizure disorders, as anyone who has familiarity with the literature about learning disabilities and hyperactivity well knows. For many people, scientific jargon is both an inconvenience and an irritant. We often wonder if these name games are really necessary, and, if so, how meaningful they are. In the case of seizure disorders, however, a compelling argument can be made for acquiring some basic information about the different types of epilepsy and for categorizing them accordingly.

Seizures differ in terms of their pattern, frequency, and duration as well as the age at which they usually begin. The prognosis and response to treatment varies depending upon the type of seizure, and, central to this discussion, the type of drug the physician selects has much to do with the kind of seizure a particular child has. Because information about seizure type can provide caregivers with some understanding of the treatment process, particularly medication, the topic of classification is discussed in some detail.

In the not too distant past, seizures were generally categorized as being either grand mal or petit mal. However, the development of more sophisticated diagnostic techniques, discovery of new antiepileptic drugs, and a more rigorous investigation of response to treatment prompted an appreciation for the various types of seizure disorders. There are at least three different approaches to classification: EEG readings, presumed cause of origin of the electrical discharge in the brain, and the outward appearance of the seizures. Livingston (1972) proposed several major types of childhood epilepsy based on EEG findings and the overt appearance of the seizures: *major motor* (tonic-clonic), *petit mal* (absence), *psychomotor* (complex partial), myoclonic epilepsy of infancy (infantile spasms), and myoclonic epilepsy of older children (Lennox-Gastaut syndrome). To facilitate research on seizure disorders, the International League Against Epilepsy has proposed a classification scheme for the epilepsies based on clinical and EEG data (Gastaut, 1970). This system is being adopted by scientists throughout the world, and the most recent version (see Commission on Classification, 1981) appears in Appendix B. Because many clinicians continue to use the more traditional terminology (Livingston, 1978a), which is also the key to all the medical literature that predates the adoption of the new classification scheme, it is essential to be fluent in both systems to understand information about seizure disorders. Therefore, in the following discussion of the various types of epilepsy, both the current and more traditional diagnostic labels are cited.

Tonic-Clonic (Grand Mal) Seizures

Approximately 80% of the children with seizure disorders have tonic-clonic seizures either as their sole epileptic manifestation or in combination with some other seizure disorder. The actual seizure consists of two phases: a *tonic* phase in which the body becomes very rigid, followed by a *clonic* phase that consists of jerking movements of the limbs (convulsions). Typically, there is a sudden loss of consciousness, the body stiffens (tonic phase), and, if standing, the child falls to the ground in the direction he or she is leaning. Breathing is suspended and the face may turn pale. This is followed by jerking movements of the body and limbs (clonic phase). During this phase of the seizure, respiration resumes and the child's breathing makes a snoring-like sound. The child may bite his or her tongue or cheek, urinate, or defecate.

If the seizure is of short duration (3 to 5 minutes), the child is usually able to resume regular activities shortly after the attack. If the seizure is long lasting (up to an hour or more), it may be followed by deep sleep. It is best to let the child sleep because attempts to awaken will not be successful. Many children, after awakening from a postseizure sleep, will exhibit any of a variety of different reactions to the seizure, including fatigue and sore muscles, nausea or headache, and behavioral changes such as irritability, restlessness, or even aggressivity. It does little good to scold or punish the child during this period. If the child's behavior is harmful to others, he or she may have to be isolated from peers until this phase of the seizure passes. Postseizure reactions may last from a few minutes to even a day or longer. The frequency of tonic-clonic seizures varies greatly among children. Some have many convulsions per day, whereas other children have only one seizure every few years.

It is not unusual for a child with tonic-clonic seizures to have a normal EEG reading. In one study of 3,101 patients with this disorder, a third had normal EEG patterns between seizures both while awake and during sleep (Livingston, 1958). There are, of course, gross changes in the EEG during the seizure as well as in the postseizure phase.

A seizure is sometimes preceded by an *aura* or brief warning that an attack will follow. In fact, the aura is actually a part of the seizure. The aura may take many forms: (a) sensory auras, which may be manifested by a "funny feeling in my stomach," dizziness, tingling sensation, or impaired vision; (b) psychic auras, examples of which are anxiety, fears, confusion, and aberrant behavior; and (c) motor auras, which include movements of the limbs, twitching, or jerking movements resulting from contractions of the skeletal muscles. Auras can be very helpful to a child by warning him or her that a seizure is imminent, thus allowing time to prevent a fall. (They may also provoke an anticipatory fear reaction.) Clearly identifiable motor auras have also been used in behavior modification programs designed to suppress seizures (e.g., Zlutnick et al., 1975). In one study, upon observing an aura, teachers and parents were able to prevent the seizure by simply holding the child and firmly saying, "Stop." Although this appears to be a promising new technique for some children with uncontrolled seizures, much research remains to be done in this area (see Mostofsky & Balaschak, 1977).

Sometimes children will have one seizure after another (*status*) or one long seizure (*prolonged*) for an extended period of time (Livingston, 1978b). These can be frightening experiences for teachers, parents, and direct care personnel in residential facilities. *Tonic-clonic status*, commonly referred to as *status epilepticus*, is defined as one complete tonic-clonic seizure after another that continues from many hours to several days. The child does not completely regain consciousness between seizures. As the seizures persist, the child becomes more comatose, dehydrated, and exhausted. Most children experiencing tonic-clonic status recover; however, death is possible. If the child regains consciousness between attacks, the condition is referred to as *serial* tonic-clonic seizures. They are frequently associated with the abrupt withdrawal of antiepileptic medication. Prolonged tonic-clonic seizures differ from tonic-clonic status in that the people experiencing the former do *not* have a recurrence of either the tonic or clonic phase after the seizure has terminated. The seizure is a prolongation of the tonic or clonic phase, usually the latter, followed by a longer than usual tonic-clonic postseizure state. Prolonged tonic-clonic seizures are associated with both diseases of the brain (e.g., meningitis and encephalitis) and epilepsy.

Studies of children and adolescents show that status epilepticus generally occurs during the first 4 years (Aicardi & Chevrie, 1970). The highest risk period is between birth and 2 years of age. Status epilepticus is often the first seizure the child ever has or occurs shortly after the onset of epilepsy. It is important to bring this type of seizure under control because it can damage the brain, leading to either transient or permanent neurological abnormality (i.e., epilepsy, mental retardation, or motor handicap). The reported prevalence of tonic-clonic status ranges from 3 to 15% among people with epilepsy, half of which experience only one episode (see Dreifuss, 1983a).

Tonic-clonic status and prolonged tonic-clonic seizures are genuine medical emergencies, and caregivers should respond accordingly. Serial tonic-clonic seizures, on the other hand, are not life threatening but should receive immediate medical attention.

Absence (Petit Mal) Seizures

Absence seizures typically manifest as a sudden, brief loss of consciousness. The child stares vacantly into space as if in a trance for several seconds, and occasionally the eyes will roll back. The actual seizure lasts from 5 to 30 seconds (average length is 10 seconds), with up to 50 or 100 "spells" per day. Absence seizures may occur in groups or "showers," particularly within a few hours after awakening in the morning. The child is often unaware that a seizure has occurred. In some cases, the staring episodes are accompanied by slight clonic movements (sudden contraction of the muscles) involving the eyebrows, eyelids, head, and/or arms. There may be rhythmic blinking of the eyes at a rate of 3 per second. Absence seizures may also be associated with *automatisms*, which are motor acts that appear purposeful but are exhibited in the wrong setting. Some examples of automatisms in children are chewing and swallowing movements, lip smacking, and mumbled speech. These are not to be confused with complex partial seizures, which may also be associated with automatisms.

Although many people are familiar with the term *petit mal*, true absence seizures are not very common. Only 2 to 3% of all individuals with epilepsy and 6 to 12% of the children with seizure disorders have petit mal spells (Currier et al., 1963). Absence seizures are truly a disorder of childhood. The most common age at onset is between 4 and 8 years, and the disorder rarely lasts beyond late adolescence. Few children with absence epilepsy are brain damaged or mentally retarded.

There is such a thing as *absence status* in which the child experiences almost continuous absence spells that may last from an hour up to a day or longer. A child who is experiencing absence status will appear inattentive and disoriented but does not stare or blink his or her eyes. Livingston et al. (1965) reported on a series of 117 patients with petit mal spells. Of the 111 who did not have evidence of brain damage prior to the onset of seizures, 7 later exhibited intellectual impairment. Six of these children had frequent episodes of absence status. Although the causal mechanisms are unknown, Livingston believed that the relationship merited consideration.

In the case of absence seizures, the EEG findings are particularly diagnostic (3 per second spike-wave forms). This abnormality is detected in most children in the resting state but can be easily induced by a few minutes of hyperventilation. Absence spells are *never* preceded by an aura or followed by a postseizure state.

Many children with absence epilepsy later develop other types of seizures, typically tonic-clonic, during adolescence. The highest incidence rates are for children between 10 and 13 years of age (Livingston et al., 1965). The probability that a child will develop another seizure disorder is influenced by both the drug regimen and the age at onset of the absence episodes. Livingston et al. compared the drug regimen for two groups of children treated for absence seizures. One group was administered a drug specifically for absence seizures, and the other group received both an antiabsence and antitonic-clonic agent. Of the group treated with only the antiabsence drug, 81% later developed tonic-clonic seizures, compared with 36% of the children receiving both drugs.

As noted, the other variable that increases the probability of developing other types of seizures is age at onset. Generally, the older the child at the time of the first absence seizure, the greater the likelihood that another seizure disorder will eventually develop. It is noteworthy that children who do develop tonic-clonic seizures subsequent to absence spells have tonic-clonic seizures that are generally not as frequent, are less severe, and are easier to control with pharmacotherapy, compared with other children with tonic-clonic epilepsy.

Partial Seizures

As previously noted, partial seizures are so named because the abnormal electrical discharges that give rise to them are localized, or confined to one area of the brain. If the electrical discharge ultimately spreads over the surface of the cortex, resulting in a tonic-clonic seizure, then it is said to be a partial seizure that is secondarily generalized. Moreover, the partial seizure may then be described as an aura. Partial seizures are classified as being either *partial seizures of elementary symptomatology* (simple) or *partial seizures of complex symptomatology* (complex). The most important feature that differentiates simple from complex partial seizures is whether or not consciousness is impaired. With simple partial seizures, consciousness is not altered. Complex partial seizures, however, are always associated with impairment, distortion, or loss of consciousness.

Simple Partial Seizures. Simple partial seizures are rare in children with the exception of *benign focal epilepsy of childhood* (with rolandic foci). This disorder is inherited and usually first begins between 5 and 10 years of age. Most seizures occur during sleep. They start with slow jerking movements of muscles on one side of the face, possibly involving the tongue, arm, and leg. This is often followed by a brief tonic-clonic seizure. The child is usually well immediately following the attack. The EEG shows abnormalities in one or both of the rolandic areas, hence the name *rolandic seizures*. The prognosis is excellent: the disorder responds well to medication and treatment can later be stopped without relapse.

Other simple partial seizures consist of jerking motor movements (*focal motor seizures*, one example of which is a Jacksonian seizure), simple sensory phenomena (e.g., abnormal sensations, flashing lights, strange smells, odd noises), autonomic phenomena (e.g., pupil dilatation, abdominal discomfort, and vomiting), altered awareness (e.g., dreamy states, flashbacks), altered mood, and cognitive phenomena (e.g., illusions, hallucinations). Children may find it very difficult to explain or describe some of these seizure-related experiences, and an abnormal EEG recording during the episode may be necessary to confirm that they are genuine epileptic phenomena.

Complex Partial Seizures. Complex partial seizures (also called *psychomotor* or *temporal lobe* seizures) are manifested in a variety of ways, including changes in behavior, mood, or sensations. These changes are associated with a clouding of consciousness and a complete or partial loss of memory of what happened during the seizure. Just about every conceivable sensory and motor aberration has been described in the literature at one time or another as a manifestation of complex partial seizures. In view of this, epileptologists have adopted more stringent criteria for the classification of complex partial seizures, limiting diagnosis to "well-defined, classical seizure patterns" usually in combination with characteristic EEG discharges (Livingston, 1972).

Before aberrant behavior is considered a manifestation of epilepsy, it must also be accompanied by abnormal EEG findings during the behavior in question. However, when the child's EEG reading is abnormal between the behavioral events that are under investigation, the diagnosis of "behavioral disorder with abnormal EEG" is assigned. In other words, a child with a behavior disorder and an abnormal *intersymptom* EEG who responds to antiepileptic medication should not, according to Livingston (1972), be assigned a diagnosis of epilepsy. Moreover, child and family expectations about improvement with medication can produce behavioral change. In general, well controlled, double-blind studies have failed to support the effectiveness of antiepileptics in the treatment of behavior disorders.

Livingston (1972) classified the complex partial seizures of children into four categories based on their outward appearance (clinical features):

1. *Arrest of activity with staring.* The staring episode is usually brief but longer than absence spells. A differential diagnosis can

be made from EEG findings. This type of complex partial seizure may last up to 5 minutes.

2. *Arrest of activity with staring followed by simple and/or complex automatisms.* Immediately following the staring episode, the child exhibits automatisms. As already discussed, these are behaviors that appear to be purposeful but are clearly out of context. Some examples are mouth movements (e.g., chewing, lip smacking, drooling, and vocalizations such as mumbling or humming). If the seizure does not terminate at this point, it may be followed by more complex automatisms. Some examples are picking at clothing or attempting to undress, handling objects, searching for things, moving around, and bizarre or abnormal behavior. Automatisms are typically stereotypic behaviors varying little from seizure to seizure. These episodes usually last a few minutes, but, as with other types of seizures, there is considerable variability in duration from one person to the next. Awareness is almost always impaired to some degree during the seizure, and there is no recollection of the attack when it is over. Complex automatisms may include aggressive and antisocial acts. Diagnosis may be quite difficult in the case of seizures that simulate behavior disorders. Livingston points out that complex partial seizures start abruptly without any apparent precipitating event, and there is usually no recollection of the attack. Behavior disorders, on the other hand, are often preceded by some triggering event, and the child usually remembers what he or she has done.

3. *Arrest of activity with staring, followed by pulling of the head and body to one side with concomitant automatisms.* Following a brief staring episode, the muscles appear to tighten as the head and body turn to one side, and an arm may extend in the direction of the turn. As stated, this rotary movement is accompanied with simple automatisms that may become complex if the seizure does not terminate immediately. The entire attack may be brief, lasting from 30 seconds to several minutes. The child typically does not remember what happened during the seizure.

4. *Psychic seizures.* These consist of a variety of sensations (e.g., hot or cold, pleasure), distorted thought (e.g., hallucinations, delusions), and changes in mood (e.g., laughing, crying). This is certainly one of the more tenuous types of epilepsy, and in the absence of clear EEG dysfunction, a diagnosis of complex partial epilepsy is questionable.

Complex partial seizures are found infrequently in children under 6 years of age. More commonly, they are exhibited in older children, adolescents, and young adults, with a prevalence of 10 to 20% in older children with seizure disorders (Gold, 1974; Livingston, 1972). It should be pointed out that, as with tonic-clonic epilepsy, complex partial seizures may be preceded by an aura and followed by a postseizure state.

Although not very common, there is such a condition as prolonged complex partial seizures. For the most part, they are unresponsive to antiepileptic drugs and are self-limiting. The child should be watched during such an episode, and measures should be taken to prevent injury.

Myoclonic Seizures

Myoclonic seizures are manifested as a twitching or jerking of skeletal muscles—usually of the head, neck, and arms. Generally, they are sudden flexor spasms. An individual muscle may contract or an entire limb may be involved. There is no apparent loss of consciousness during the attack. These seizures may occur a few at a time or in a series, one after another. What the seizure will look like depends upon the age of the child and position of the body when the seizure begins. A variety of different seizure disorders are subsumed under the label myoclonic epilepsy. Livingston (1972) identified two types of myoclonic epilepsy based upon the age at which the seizures first began: infancy versus early childhood.

The earliest emerging myoclonic epilepsy is *infantile spasms*. It develops during the first year, usually between the third and ninth month. If the child is lying down, seizures may take the following form: flexion of the head forward, outward thrust of the arms, and flexion of the thighs up on the abdomen. It may be quite difficult to discriminate these seizures from normal infant activity or colic. The seizures are very brief, lasting a few seconds, and some infants may have up to 100 seizures per day. Seizures are exhibited in rapid succession, lasting from 1 or 2 minutes with no apparent loss of consciousness. If the infant is sitting, the spell may consist of a sudden forward jerk of the head accompanied by an outward thrust of the arms (head dropping or head nodding spells). Infantile spasms generally abate between 3 and 4 years of age. Unfortunately, they are often replaced by other types of seizure disorders, particularly the Lennox-Gastaut syndrome.

A second form of myoclonic epilepsy is *Lennox-Gastaut syndrome*. This disorder develops after 2 years of age, usually between

3 and 7 years. The seizure pattern in the sitting position is similar to that described for infants who are able to sit. The head suddenly jerks forward (occasionally backward), and the arms are thrust outward. If the child is holding an object, it may drop from his or her hands or, in some cases, may be thrown across the room. Again, these are referred to as "head-nodding" or "head-dropping" spells by some clinicians. In the standing position, the sudden flexor spasm, often associated with an outward thrust of the arms, frequently results in a vehement fall forward. However, the child is usually able to get up right after the attack. Such falls often result in lacerations of the forehead, nose, and chin. To prevent such injuries, the child can wear protective head gear similar to a football helmet. Such attacks usually occur on a daily basis. Although each individual spell may last only a few seconds, they often occur in groups or showers lasting several minutes.

Youngsters with Lennox-Gastaut syndrome often experience a mixture of seizures. They include sudden falls that may or may not be preceded by violent jerks (drop seizures), absence seizures that are characterized by a cessation of motion (akinetic), blinking of the eyelids and upward movement of the eyes, head-nodding seizures, sagging (atonic) or loss of posture (astatic), and tonic-clonic seizures. The attacks may be so frequent that the child fears walking alone.

Because few followup studies have been conducted on children with myoclonic epilepsy, little can be said about how the disorder changes during adolescence and adulthood. Livingston (1972) found that many of the children whose seizures began in infancy continued to experience them into childhood. Niedermeyer (1974) reported the seizure pattern may be quite irregular, making the evaluation of drug effectiveness difficult. The older child may have a complete cessation of attacks for several years. With increasing age the atonic and myoclonic seizures generally cease, only to be replaced by tonic-clonic (often nocturnal) and/or complex partial seizures (Dreifuss, 1983a).

The EEG of infants with infantile spasms "gives the impression of nearly total disorganization of cortical voltage regulation" (Livingston, 1974, p. 543). The actual EEG pattern is referred to as hypsarrhythmia. This pattern changes to modified hypsarrhythmia as the child gets older.

Most infants diagnosed as having infantile spasms show clear evidence of brain damage prior to the onset of seizures, and almost all are severely mentally and/or motorically retarded. For the older children, the incidence of specific brain damage prior to the onset of seizures and the severity of mental retardation is much less than for the infants. The earlier the onset of these seizures, the poorer the prognosis in terms of mental retardation and motor development. "It has been our experience that the most serious hazard of childhood myoclonic epilepsy is not the seizure *per se*, but the associated mental retardation" (Livingston, 1972, p. 84).

A third type of myoclonic epilepsy is found in children who experience only myoclonic jerks. Mental retardation is rare, and the prognosis is very favorable.

Benign juvenile myoclonic epilepsy is yet another type of myoclonic seizure disorder (see Asconapé & Penry, 1984). Its onset is usually during adolescence and is characterized by myoclonic jerks, which usually occur on awakening. Most youths who seek medical attention for this condition also experience tonic-clonic seizures, and approximately one third have a history of absence seizures. Teenagers with benign myoclonic epilepsy are typically of normal intellectual ability. EEG findings provide important diagnostic information.

In addition to these four types of myoclonic epilepsy, it is believed that other forms exist as well (see, for example, Jeavons, 1977). Because these other types of myoclonic epilepsy are either very rare or not widely recognized in the clinical literature, they have not been described here.

Febrile Seizures

There are a number of disorders that appear similar to epilepsy because they involve a loss of consciousness, are episodic in nature, or involve convulsive body movements. Febrile seizures are one such disorder, and, because these attacks are relatively common among young children, they are included in this discussion. The term *febrile* means fever, and *febrile* seizure simply refers to seizures associated with a febrile illness.

Based on several studies of a large number of young children exhibiting seizures in association with fever, Livingston (1972) identified two disorders: *simple febrile seizures* and *epileptic seizures precipitated by fever*. Simple febrile seizures usually have their onset between 9 and 18 months of age and rarely begin after the child is 5 years old. They are associated with childhood illnesses that do not involve the brain, such as upper respiratory infections, otitis media (inflammation of the middle ear), and pneumonia (Nelson & Ellenberg, 1978). The seizures are always generalized (usually tonic-clonic) and are brief, lasting no longer than a few minutes. Typically, the child has only one seizure per illness, and it occurs between 2 to 6 hours after the onset of the fever. The prognosis for simple febrile seizures is excellent. Most children only have one to three seizures per year and the disorder rarely lasts beyond 6 years of age. Simple febrile seizures are relatively common. In one massive followup study of approximately 54,000 children, it was reported that 3.5% of the white children and 4.2% of the black children experienced at least one febrile seizure (Nelson & Ellenberg, 1978).

Epileptic seizures associated with fever (atypical febrile seizures) are quite different from simple febrile seizures in terms of treatment and prognosis. According to Livingston (1972), the diagnosis of atypical febrile seizure is made if the child has one or more of the following: prolonged seizures, focal convulsions of any duration, febrile convulsions after the age of 5, and EEG findings that are characteristic of epilepsy. The prognosis for children with epileptic seizures associated with fever is similar to other children with epilepsy.

General Comments

Although this classification scheme may create the impression that children with seizure disorders fall neatly into a given category, such is not the case. Children may have more than one type of seizure disorder during the same period of time, or one form of epilepsy may be followed by another later in life. As noted previously, absence seizures in childhood may be followed by tonic-clonic seizures in adolescence or early adulthood. Prevalence figures for mixed epilepsy (more than one kind of seizure) vary ranging from 40 to 60% in the people with seizure disorders (Epilepsy Foundation of America, 1975).

Unfortunately, verbal descriptions of seizures are a far from satisfactory means of education. To give caregivers a better idea of what the different types of seizures look like, I have used several films that are of value in this regard. One film, *Modern Concepts of Epilepsy* (Ayerst Laboratories) is now dated but is quite useful in its graphic presentations of a variety of seizures. Another film that features Dr. Livingston, *Diagnosis and Medical Management of Epileptic Seizures* (Ayerst Laboratories), was developed to train pediatricians about epilepsy. With appropriate preparation, it is also an excellent film for graduate level teacher-training programs, as is *Complex Partial Seizures* (Geigy Pharmaceuticals). A number of other films about epilepsy have been made, and information about their content and availability can be obtained from the Epilepsy Foundation of America.

PSEUDOEPILEPTIC SEIZURES

Pseudoepileptic seizures or *pseudoseizures* are seizurelike behaviors, but they are not true seizures because the are not associated with an abnormal EEG (during the "seizure") or a true state of altered consciousness. They are more common in adolescents and females than in prepubertal children or males and in children with a history of epilepsy compared with those who do not have such a background (see Goodyer, 1985). Accurate diagnosis of pseudoseizures is very important for at least two reasons: One, pseudoseizures should be treated with behavioral interventions (see Williams & Mostofsky, 1982), not medication; two, failure to diagnose pseudoseizures for what they are may lead to excessive medication and/or unnecessary multiple-drug therapy.

Psuedoseizures can be very difficult to diagnose. In a paper describing a series of case studies, Goodyer (1985) noted three clues that alerted medical staff to the possibility of pseudoseizures: marked anxiety, hyperventilation prior to symtpom onset, and lack of *postictal phenomena* (altered state or behavior following seizure). Sophisticated EEG procedures that permit concurrent recording of behavior and EEG or that allow freedom of movement in natural settings (see Stores, 1985) are making the task of diagnosis less difficult.

SEIZURE MANAGEMENT

For parents, teachers, direct care personnel in residential facilities, and many other care providers, a tonic-clonic seizure can be a frightening experience. Because there have been conflicting opinions about how best to care for a person during a grand mal seizure, some confusion may exist as to what is the proper thing to do. The following steps should be taken during the course of a seizure:

1. Remove any objects that the child may strike during the clonic phase (jerking movements) of the seizure.
2. Loosen restricting clothing.
3. Turn the child on his or her side. (This will allow saliva and vomitus to flow out of the mouth instead of being aspirated.)
4. Do not try to restrain the child's movements during the active (tonic-clonic) phase of the seizure.
5. Do not try to move the child during the active phase of the seizure.
6. Do not insert any objects into the child's mouth.

In case there is any confusion regarding the last point, the following quote from Lombroso (1974) is quite emphatic:

> Most convulsive seizures are self-limiting events terminating on their own accord before specific medical treatment need or can be rendered. For these, positioning to prevent aspiration of excessive secretions and vomitus and prevention of self-injuries is generally sufficient. Prying open clenched teeth for the insertion of time-honored tongue blades, pencils or fingers has no place in modern medicine. These maneuvers are useless in the prevention of tongue biting (that will have occurred at the onset of the initial tonic phase), but may actually be harmful by dislodging loose teeth, and by initiating nociceptive stimuli that reflexly can prolong the tonic phase. Likewise excessive restraining of convulsing patients may facilitate bone injuries. (p. 536)

Because there is some disagreement among epileptologists regarding the prevention of tongue and cheek biting (Livingston, 1978b), the following procedure is suggested for school personnel. In those *rare* cases in which the physician recommends than an object be placed in the child's mouth to prevent self-injury, specific instructions should be obtained from the doctor on how this situation should be handled and by whom. Simply asking the parents if any special procedures are required to keep the child from hurting himself or herself during a seizure can allay fears about what the school should do.

Many children will be able to resume classroom activities shortly after the seizure. However, some youngsters lapse into a deep sleep. Attempts to awaken them are futile, and they should be allowed to sleep. Upon awakening, the child may be confused, afraid, upset, or exhibit unusual behavior. Scolding is of little value. If the child's postseizure behavior is self-injurious or harmful to others, appropriate measures must be taken. The same holds true for complex partial seizures if automatisms manifest as behavior disorders. Fortunately, attitudes about epilepsy have changed over the last half century, and attempts to conceal the disorder are not as pervasive as they once were. Caregivers should definitely be informed of the seizure disorder even if medication keeps the attacks completely under control. The awareness that a child has epilepsy may cause some apprehension for school personnel and other care providers, especially if they are not informed about the type of seizure and degree of seizure control with medication or have not been in such a situation before (Force, 1965). To repeat, the easiest thing to do is simply ask the parents or primary care personnel what they do when their child has a seizure.

Unfortunately, space constraints do not permit a discussion of the psychosocial aspects of epilepsy. It must be emphasized, however, that reactions to a seizure greatly influence how peers and other adults respond to the child with epilepsy. In the case of a child with uncontrolled seizures, the teacher, for example, can explain the disorder to the class (if necessary, in the child's absence), and even use classroom activities that sensitize students to the needs of exceptional children. It is the unexpectedness of the seizure and alarmed reaction of the teacher and peers that makes the situation tragic. Much of this can be avoided with a little preparation. Many teachers have shared with me anecdotes of how tonic-clonic seizures can be made quite uneventful with appropriate peer sensitization and personal conversations with the epileptic child.

The probability of encountering children with uncontrolled seizures is greatly influenced by the educational setting. In regular elementary and secondary schools in which fewer than 1% of the students are treated for epilepsy, the probability is low. Considering that at least 50% of such children are seizure-free if they take their medication regularly, a tonic-clonic seizure at school may be a rare event. Force (1965), however, reported that a third of the nonspecial education teachers in his survey had witnessed a seizure at school, as did over 80% of the special education teachers. In another study, over half of the special education teachers had direct experience with tonic-clonic seizures in their classrooms for mentally retarded children (Gadow, 1978). For special education settings, the proportion of children treated for seizure disorders who have seizures at school ranges from 27% in early childhood classes to 41% in programs for trainable mentally retarded children (Gadow, 1977; 1978). It is likely that the recent emphasis on deinstitutionalization, mainstreaming, and least restrictive placement will bring many more people into contact with children and adolescents who have seizures.

MEDICATION FOR DIFFERENT TYPES OF SEIZURES

By far the most common treatment for seizure disorders is drug therapy. Generally speaking, antiepileptic drugs are capable of rendering 50% of the children with epilepsy seizure-free. Another 25% have fewer and less-severe seizures, leaving approximately 15% of the treatment population who are not helped with medication. Unfortunately, of the children with *intractable* (uncontrollable) seizures, only a small percentage are good candidates for surgery, a treatment rarely employed with children. Unless the exact location of the abnormal electrical discharge (focus) can be identified, surgery is often impractical. Even when surgery is successful, antiepileptic medication must continue to be administered. Other types of treatment are sometimes used. For example, a special diet may be quite helpful for the child with myoclonic epilepsy. A relatively new surgical technique involves placing inside the body a small electrical device that stimulates the cerebellum, thus inhibiting seizures (Cooper et al., 1976). As noted previously, there is now much interest in investigating psychological treatments for controlling seizures such as psychotherapy, behavior modification, and biofeedback (Mostofsky & Balaschak, 1977). Although some children may benefit from nondrug treatments, this section focuses on medication, in keeping with the orientation of this text.

Bromides were found to be useful agents in the treatment of epilepsy in 1853, and phenobarbital was introduced in 1912 (see Livingston, 1972). For many years, these were the only drugs that were truly effective in the control of seizures. Because bromides and phenobarbital often produced sedation (drowsiness, lethargy) at the same dosages required to control attacks, they were far from satisfactory for all people with epilepsy. In a paper published in 1937, Putnam and Merritt observed that little progress had been made to develop more effective antiepileptics. They also reported that Dilantin (phenytoin), among other drugs they were investigating, had anticonvulsant properties in laboratory animals. Shortly thereafter, Dilantin was found to be quite effective in controlling tonic-clonic attacks but had little effect on absence seizures (Merritt & Putnam, 1938). It was not until 1945 that the first effective antiabsence drug, Tridione (trimethadione) was discussed in the literature (Lennox, 1945). Today there are hundreds of drugs known to have antiepileptic properties; however, less than two dozen are used with any frequency, and three or four drugs account for most of all medication used in the management of these disorders. Before discussing the effects of Dilantin, Tridione, and other more recently developed agents, it should be emphasized that many antiepileptic drugs are truly miracles of modern pharmacological research.

The commonly prescribed drugs for the control of seizures consist primarily of five groups of antiepileptics (see Table 2–1). The drugs within each group have similar properties. A sixth category of agents, made up of psychotropic and assorted other drugs, have antiepileptic properties but are also used for the treatment of other disorders.

As previously stated, the various types of seizure disorders respond most favorably to different types of antiepileptics. In Table 2–2 drugs are listed in order of preference for four major groups of

Table 2-1. Antiepileptic Drugs Grouped According to Similarities in Chemical Structure

Barbiturates	**Benzodiazepines**
Gemonil (metharbital)	Clonopin (clonazepam)
Mebaral (mephobarbital)	Tranxene (clorazepate)
Mysoline (primidone)	Valium (diazepam)
phenobarbital	
	Other Drugs
Hydantoinates	ACTH (corticotropin) and
Dilantin (phenytoin)	corticosteroids
Mesantoin (mephenytoin)	Atabrine (quinacrine)
Peganone (ethotoin)	bromides
	Depakene (valproic acid)
Succinimides	Dexedrine (dextroamphetamine)
Celontin (methsuximide)	Diamox (acetazolamide)
Milontin (phensuximide)	Phenurone (phenacemide)
Zarontin (ethosuximide)	Tegretol (carbamazepine)
Oxazolidinediones	
Paradione (paramethadione)	
Tridione (trimethadione)	

seizure disorders. This selection and ranking of drugs is based upon Livingston's (1972) research on the safety and efficacy of these agents.

Tonic-Clonic (Grand Mal) Seizures

Phenobarbital is the drug of first choice in the treatment of tonic-clonic seizures. It is both the least toxic and least expensive of the major antiepileptics. There is, however, disagreement about the selection of phenobarbital as the first agent to be tried. Some experts feel it should be Dilantin because it is a more powerful drug. Livingston (1972) believed that the large number of side effects associated with Dilantin made it less desirable and that it should not be recommended for treatment in infants, adolescent females, and children undergoing orthodontal care. The rationales for these exclusions were: (a) it is difficult to evaluate side effects in infants; (b) the possibility of excessive growth of body hair and gum tissue makes it undesirable for females; and (c) the growth of gum tissue interferes with orthodontal treatments. Because phenobarbital may cause hyperactivity or irritability as a side effect, Mebaral (mephobarbital) is listed as a possible alternative. Mysoline (primidone) is the second most preferred agent for the treatment of tonic-clonic epilepsy. It is noteworthy that one of the metabolites of Mysoline is phenobarbital. Diamox (acetazolamide) may be helpful as an

Table 2–2. Drugs Currently Used at the Samuel Livingston Epilepsy Diagnostic and Treatment Center for the Control of Epileptic Seizures*

Tonic-Clonic	Absence	Complex Partial	Infantile Spasms	Myoclonic	Lennox-Gastaut Syndrome
PHENOBARBITAL (Mebaral)[1]	ZARONTIN	TEGRETOL	ACTH and CORTICOSTE-ROIDS	Valium	KETOGENIC DIET[5]
MYSOLINE	DEPAKENE	Mysoline		Bromide	ACTH and CORTICOSTE-ROIDS
DILANTIN	Tridione[3]	Dilantin		Clonopin	
Tegretol	Paradione[3]	Mesantoin[2]		Depakene	
Bromide (for young children)	Celontin	Phenurone[2]			
Peganone	Milontin				
Gemonil	Dexedrine				
Mesantoin[2]	Atabrine[4]				
Dexedrine (for sleep seizures)					
Diamox (for menstrual seizures)					

Note: From *Comprehensive Management of Epilepsy in Infancy, Childhood and Adolescence* (p. 194) by S. Livingston, 1972, Springfield, IL: Charles C Thomas. Copyright 1972 by Charles C Thomas, Publisher. Adapted by permission.

* Arranged in order of our preference, based on relative efficacy and toxicity.

[1] We use this drug almost exclusively as a substitute barbiturate for patients whose seizures are benefited by dosages of phenobarbital that produce side reactions, such as marked drowsiness or hyperactivity.

[2] These drugs possess potent anticonvulsant properties, but because of pronounced toxicity, they should be prescribed only to patients whose seizures are refractory to all other antiepileptic agents.

[3] These drugs are very effective in controlling absence spells, but they appear to be potent teratogens. All other antiabsence agents should be given an adequate trial before prescribing these drugs to females of child-bearing age.

[4] Atabrine is effective in the treatment of some cases, but its value is limited because it causes a yellowish discoloration of the skin in most patients.

[5] The ketogenic diet is included because of its exceptional value in controlling this form of epilepsy.

adjunct for the management of tonic-clonic seizures associated with menstruation.

Tegretol (carbamazepine) is an effective medication for the management of tonic-clonic seizures (e.g., Huf & Schain, 1980), and for many clinicians, it is the drug of first choice (e.g., Schain, 1983). Tegretol's popularity stems from the fact that, unlike phenobarbital, it does not cause hyperactivity or mental impairments; and unlike Dilantin, it is not associated with cosmetic side effects that may lead to psychological adjustment problems. Because brain-damaged and mentally retarded children are more susceptible to the sedative effects of antiepileptic drugs, its use with these populations may be particularly beneficial (see Schain, 1983).

Depakene (valproic acid) is also considered to be an effective agent for the treatment of tonic-clonic seizures. There are two situations for which it is purportedly most useful (Dreifuss, 1983b). The first is for children who have both absence and tonic-clonic seizures. Second is the treatment of *reflex-induced* tonic-clonic seizures. Such seizures are precipitated by an environmental stimulus such as a flashing light, visual patterns, and certain sounds (e.g., a police car siren).

Prolonged tonic-clonic seizures, serial tonic-clonic seizures, and tonic-clonic status can be treated with intravenous injections of Valium, paraldehyde, or barbiturates in an attempt to terminate the seizure (Livingston, 1978b). In general, the longer these seizures last, the more difficult they are to stop. To repeat, a child experiencing any of these three types of prolonged seizures should receive immediate medical attention. Tonic-clonic status, in particular, is a serious medical emergency.

Absence (Petit Mal) Seizures

The drug of first choice for the treatment of absence seizures is Zarontin (ethosuximide). It was first reported to be an effective agent for this type of seizure in 1958 (Zimmerman & Burgemeister, 1958). Although extremely effective in the control of absence seizures, it is of little importance for other types of attacks. Because a high percentage of children with absence epilepsy develop other kinds of seizures later on, Livingston (1972) recommended the following regimen: Drug treatment should be initiated with phenobarbital as a prophylactic measure against the development of tonic-clonic seizures. The physician observes if phenobarbital is well tolerated in terms of side effects and to see that it does not increase the frequency of petit mal spells. If phenobarbital is unsatisfactory, other antitonic-clonic agents (Mysoline, Mebaral) are tried. Because

Dilantin may exacerbate absence attacks, it is tried only after other drugs have failed. Once the child has adjusted to the antitonic-clonic agent (after about 1 month of treatment), the antiabsence drug is started. Zarontin should be tried first. If this fails to control the absence seizures, then other medication must be attempted (see Table 2–2). Drugs for both the control of tonic-clonic and absence seizures are maintained until the child has been seizure-free for at least 4 years. If the EEG no longer shows the characteristic absence pattern, the dosage of the antiabsence drug is gradually reduced over a 6 to 12 month period. The tonic-clonic agent is continued until the age of 14. If the child has not developed tonic-clonic epilepsy by then, the dosage of the tonic-clonic drug is reduced over a 1 year period, and treatment is terminated. Although Livingston et al. (1965) reported findings that support the clinical utility of this procedure, it is not known if it has been widely adopted. Many neurologists appear to use monotherapy with an antiabsence agent unless the child is actually experiencing another type of seizure (Sato, 1983).

Depakene, approved by the FDA in 1978, is the most recent addition to the list of drugs proven effective in the control of petit mal spells (Gram et al., 1977; Jeavons & Clark, 1974), and it is considered by some to be the drug of first choice for the treatment of absence seizures (e.g., Sherwin, 1983). Depakene was shown to be equally effective as Zarontin in the control of absence seizures (Sato et al., 1982), but for many Zarontin remains the preferred medication (e.g., Dreifuss, 1983a; Livingston 1978a). When neither Zarontin nor Depakene produces adequate seizure control, a combination of the two drugs has proven effective.

Clonopin (clonazepam) is another powerful antiabsence drug (Mikkelsen et al., 1976). Unfortunately, a high rate of side effects has greatly limited its use. Also, tolerance often develops during the course of treatment. When adverse reactions do prompt drug withdrawal, medication should be terminated gradually to prevent the occurrence of a rebound effect (a tonic-clonic seizure).

Other antiepileptic drugs are also recommended for the treatment of absence epilepsy. Millichap (1972), for example, reports that Diamox is equally as effective as Zarontin and causes fewer side effects. However, some clinicians report that Diamox produces only temporary seizure control in many cases (Livingston, 1978a).

Myoclonic Seizures

Because the severe forms of myoclonic epilepsy are often unresponsive to medication, this disorder with its concomitant mental retardation will be a trying experience for the family. Huttenlocher et al. (1971), for example, described the case of an 11-year-old girl with myoclonic seizures who responded favorably to a special diet. However, repeated falls during childhood "led to widespread scarring of the face and chronic ulceration . . . of the skin over her forehead . . . . Uncontrolled seizures made school attendance impossible. She became withdrawn and self-conscious due to her disfigured face" (p. 1101–1102). The following quote from Niedermeyer (1974) aptly describes the seriousness of the situation from the standpoint of the physician:

> Desperate parents sometimes ask for *neurosurgical treatment* but in view of the widespread EEG abnormalities, the neurosurgeon will have to resist, in most instances, the parental pressure to operate. *Institutionalization* is very frequently the result of the severe mental defects which may lay an unbearable burden on the life of an otherwise healthy family. (p. 92)

Obviously such a situation presents a number of risk-to-benefit questions about treatment itself. As Niedermeyer (1974) put it:

> Should the physician give medication at all? I feel one cannot negate this question, especially because of the psychological impact of total therapeutic passivity on parents and relatives. It may be wise to change medication from time to time, according to general rules of such changes. . . . A dramatic struggle for a pharmacological enforcement of seizure-freedom has to be strictly avoided; these attempts always lead to drug toxicity and enhancement of mental dullness. (p. 92)

Of all the types of epilepsy, infantile spasms and the Lennox-Gastaut syndrome carry the worst prognosis in terms of seizure suppression. In infants and young children, ACTH (corticotropin) and corticosteroids may be effective in the control of seizures (Livingston, 1972). However, the relapse rate is high, and there is no beneficial effect on mental performance. The best results are obtained with infants (less than a year old) when treatment begins soon after the onset of seizures.

Livingston (1978a) considered Valium to be the preferred drug in the treatment of Lennox-Gastaut syndrome and for infantile spasms when steroid treatment is not started shortly after the onset of seizures. Unfortunately, the beneficial effects of Valium are often short-lived. After a few months of treatment, children typically develop a tolerance for the drug's seizure controlling properties.

At the present time, Depakene is probably considered the drug of first choice in the treatment of myoclonic epilepsy (DeVivo, 1983; Dreifuss, 1983a) and is often used in combination with other antiepileptic drugs when tonic-clonic seizures are also present. Unfortunately, it appears as if this very same group of epileptic children are also at greatest risk for the adverse effects of Depakene therapy both from the standpoint of drug interactions, behavioral toxicity, and serious somatic side effects.

Clonopin is also effective in the treatment of myoclonic epilepsy (e.g., Fazio et al., 1973), and, like Valium, is a benzodiazepine. Clonopin was approved by the FDA in 1975. Although its initial appearance was associated with much enthusiasm, it has fallen into disfavor for the treatment of this seizure disorder to bothersome side effects (e.g., drowsiness, behavioral change), development of tolerance, and rebound effects (tonic-clonic seizures) upon dosage reduction (Dreifuss, 1983a).

The most effective drug for the treatment of benign juvenile myoclonic epilepsy is reported to be Depakene (see Asconapé & Penry, 1984).

Livingston (1972) has been a strong advocate of the ketogenic diet in the control of myoclonic seizures, especially in children between 2 and 5 years of age. Briefly, the diet prescribes that the amount (in grams) of fat consumed must be at least four times greater than the amount (in grams) of carbohydrates and protein combined. Although there are a number of problems inherent in this regimen, it has proved to be quite effective for many children with myoclonic (and tonic-clonic) seizures. In some cases, however, the benefits of the ketogenic diet are short-lived, with a recurrence of seizures after several months of treatment. Two additional benefits of the diet are (a) a marked tranquilizing effect on epileptic children who are also hyperactive (even in the absence of seizure control) and (b) an avoidance of the side effects associated with antiepileptic drugs. The reader is referred to Livingston (1972, pp. 378–405) for a more detailed discussion.

In recent years, interest has been generated about the use of medium chain triglycerides (MCT) to provide the necessary fat content in the ketogenic diet (e.g., Huttenlocher et al., 1971; Signore, 1973; Trauner, 1985). Advocates maintain that the use of MCT permits a more palatable diet without loss of seizure control. Others, however, have not found the MCT diet to be as effective as the ketogenic diet in controlling myoclonic seizures (Livingston et al., 1977).

Partial Seizures

The drug of choice in the treatment of partial epilepsy (benign focal epilepsy of childhood, simple partial seizures, and complex partial seizures) is Tegretol (carbamazepine). It was approved by the FDA for use in the treatment of epilepsy in 1974. Because Tegretol is capable of *autoinduction* (it stimulates production of microsomal enzymes for its own biotransformation), the dosage may have to be increased during long-term therapy. Although it is considered superior to other agents in the control of complex partial seizures (Livingston, 1978a), some clinicians report Dilantin and Mysoline are equally effective (e.g., Livingston et al., 1978; Rodin et al., 1976). Two additional drugs that are effective for complex partial seizures, particularly when used in combination with other antiepileptic agents, are Depakene and Tranxene (clorazepate) (see Dreifuss, 1983a).

Nocturnal (Sleep) Seizures

Nocturnal seizures typically occur soon after falling asleep or shortly before or after the usual time of awakening. These seizures are usually difficult to control with standard antiepileptic drugs (phenobarbital, Dilantin, Mysoline). However, Dexedrine (dextroamphetamine) has been used successfully in the management of nocturnal seizures, especially those that occur shortly after falling asleep (Livingston & Pauli, 1975). It is noteworthy that after treating 10,000 epileptics with amphetamines, particularly Dexedrine, Livingston reported these drugs are remarkably free of side effects. He did not encounter drug addiction in a single case!

Febrile Seizures

Perhaps one of the most debated topics in pharmacotherapy for seizure disorders is the treatment of simple febrile seizures. The source of the problem has a lot to do with the definition of febrile seizure. Because not all researchers use the same criteria, children with epileptic seizures precipitated by fever (atypical febrile seizures) may be included in treatment samples. Another problem is parent compliance with drug therapy (i.e., it is difficult to be certain if the treated group is really receiving medication). Livingston (1972) argued that drug treatment for simple febrile seizures is neither necessary nor effective. Such seizures appear to be unresponsive to continuous antiepileptic drug treatment (e.g., with phenobarbital), and giving the child phenobarbital at the onset of a fever is of little value because the seizure is often the first indication to the parent that the child has a fever. He further noted that administering phenobarbital and aspirin at the onset of a fever may be useful because "it provides the parents with 'something to do' and may relieve some of their anxiety'' (1972, p. 30).

Wolf et al. (1977) also found that when phenobarbital is given intermittently, it is no more effective in preventing febrile seizures than when no medication is administered. In contrast to Livingston, however, they found that continuous (daily) treatment with phenobarbital did significantly reduce the occurrence of febrile seizures. The major problems they encountered with prescribing phenobarbital for use on a daily basis were parental resistance and failure to give medication regularly and drug-induced hyperactivity (see section on side effects). Attempts have been made to identify children who are at risk for developing epilepsy subsequent to febrile seizures (Nelson & Ellenberg, 1978). However, it is not known if continuous treatment with phenobarbital after the onset of febrile seizures will prevent the eventual development of epilepsy in high risk children. In general, "there is no empiric evidence that chronic treatment with anticonvulsant medication influences, positively or negatively, the long-term prognosis of children with febrile seizures" (Nelson & Ellenberg, 1978, p. 726).

Treatment of epileptic seizures precipitated by fever, however, should be initiated immediately and monitored like any other seizure disorder. Considering the side effects associated with Dilantin, phenobarbital should be employed first in attempting to control seizures in infants. Depakene and Mysoline have also been reported to be effective for "complicated" febrile seizures and simple febrile seizures associated with risk factors (Herranz et al., 1984).

General Comments

In actual clinical practice, physicians may use drugs other than those employed by Livingston in the treatment of certain types of seizure disorders. When frequently used agents fail to control seizures, other more powerful (and possibly more toxic) drugs may have to be administered, or the physician may have no other alternative than to try drugs with known antiepileptic effects but not specifically approved by the FDA for the treatment of epilepsy. New and experimental drugs are typically first used with people whose seizures cannot be controlled with conventional medication.

SIDE EFFECTS OF ANTIEPILEPTIC DRUGS

Unwanted antiepileptic drug reactions can be classified according to: (a) intoxication due to high levels of the drug in the blood, (b) common side effects that occur at normal dosages, and (c) idiosyncratic reactions that are unrelated to dosage (Kutt & Louis, 1972). This discussion of side effects focuses primarily on drug-induced behavioral changes that impair performance and changes in bodily function that are observable to care providers.

Barbiturates

The barbiturates (phenobarbital, Mysoline, and Mebaral) are among the most frequently prescribed drugs for epilepsy. Phenobarbital is the least likely to produce serious side effects of all the antiepileptics. Livingston (1972) commented after treating 15,000 patients with this drug, many for long periods of time, that "the only significant untoward reactions we have observed in our patients are drowsiness, hyperactivity and excitation simulating the hyperkinetic syndrome and an occasional rash" (p. 174).

Drowsiness is a common side effect of phenobarbital, but in many children this reaction diminishes within a few weeks after the onset of treatment. If drowsiness persists, the physician may attempt to counteract it with a stimulant drug (e.g., Ritalin or Dexedrine). If this in unsuccessful, a decision will have to be made whether or not to select another antiepileptic medication. The pervasiveness of drowsiness with phenobarbital treatment among children with seizure disorders is demonstrated in three separate surveys. In a study of 101 children receiving antiepileptics in early childhood special education programs (Gadow, 1982), teachers rated 36% as being more drowsy or sleepy than their peers. The figure for 241 mentally retarded public school children on medication for seizures was 37% (Gadow, 1982). A survey conducted by the National Epilepsy League (Pietsch, 1977) found that 35% of the children on medication were considered drowsy by their parents. It should be emphasized that some children *may* simulate drowsiness as a device for manipulating both parents and teachers. Nevertheless, the consistency of these results across treatment populations indicates that this side effect has educational implications for a large number of children treated with antiepileptic medication.

Another side effect of phenobarbital in children is behavior disorders, which may be manifested as irritability, aggressivity, excitability, overactivity, and/or hyperactivity. This has been documented in the clinical literature for many years (e.g., Cutts & Jasper, 1939; Lindsley & Henry, 1941). Livingston (1972) estimated that 15 to 20% of the children he treated with phenobarbital experienced this type of reaction. Similarly, Gadow (1977) found that 20% of the preschoolers taking phenobarbital for epilepsy exhibited behavior problems as a result of medication. The prevalence of drug induced hyperactivity, aggressivity, and irritability in children treated for febrile seizures was 25% in one study (Thorn, 1975) and 42% in another (Wolf & Forsythe, 1978). In some cases, the behavior disorder is severe and becomes an even greater problem than the seizures. Wolf and Forsythe (1978) reported that phenobarbital treatment had to be discontinued in half of the children who developed this reaction. They also noted a relationship between this side effect and preexisting behavioral disturbance. Only 20% of the children whose behavior was normal before seizures began developed a behavioral disturbance on phenobarbital compared with 80% for those who exhibited behavior disorders prior to the onset of seizures. In the latter group, phenobarbital seems to aggravate the situation. However, not everyone agrees that this side effect is more common in behavior-disordered children (Livingston, 1976). Phenobarbital-induced behavioral disturbances are not dose-related but rather represent a specific sensitivity to the drug. Livingston (1978b) suggested that the physician should first see if Ritalin or Dexedrine is effective in controlling the behavior disorder. If unsuccessful, phenobarbital should be gradually replaced with Mebaral. If the behavior problems still do not abate, Mebaral should be substituted with Mysoline.

Skin rashes are rare with phenobarbital. In general, when anti-epileptics do produce skin reactions, the physician discontinues the offending agent and substitutes another drug (Livingston, 1978b). Dosage reduction usually does not help because skin reactions are due to a specific sensitivity to the drug.

Compared with phenobarbital, Mebaral is much less likely to produce drowsiness or a hyperactivity reaction (Livingston, 1972).

The primary side effect of Mysoline is drowsiness, particularly when the drug is first taken. If the reaction is persistent, treatment may have to be discontinued. Other possible side effects (which usually disappear within a few weeks) are dizziness, *diplopia* (double vision), and *ataxia* (a staggered walk with a wide base, making a child appear as if he or she is drunk). *Dysarthria* (slurred speech), *nystagmus* (rapid, involuntary movement of the eyeball), and headaches are also side effects associated with either early treatment or overmedication. Measlelike rashes are occasionally reported with Mysoline treatment.

Hydantoinates

Dilantin and Mesantoin (mephenytoin) have very powerful antiepileptic properties, but they also are associated with a wide variety of side effects. Peganone (ethotoin) is the least toxic and the least potent. Dilantin is considered to be a relatively safe drug when properly administered and can be prescribed for long periods of time without any apparent discomfort (Livingston, 1972). Because Dilantin typically does not produce drowsiness, its discovery was met with much enthusiasm.

Several disturbances are associated with overmedication (Dilantin *intoxication*). These include ataxia, diplopia, nystagmus, and dysarthria. However, these side effects can usually be managed with dosage reduction. Unfortunately, the dosage that is effective in controlling seizures also frequently borders on the level that produces intoxication.

Excessive growth of gum tissue (*gingival hyperplasia*) is also quite common, occurring in approximately 40% of those treated with Dilantin. Visually, the gums enlarge and, in severe cases, they grow over the surface area of the teeth, creating a mulberrylike appearance. Food particles and other irritants lodge in the gums, causing them to redden or have a bluish cast. Meticulous oral hygiene and gum massage are often stressed. Although this can alleviate inflammation due to food particles, it does not slow down or lessen the growth of gum tissue (Livingston & Livingston, 1973). This reaction usually starts 2 to 3 months into treatment and is more common among children than adults. Livingston (1972) reported that the growth of gum tissue is *not* dose-related, but there is some disagreement (Little et al., 1975). The gums return to normal 3 to 12 months after medication is stopped, depending upon the severity of tissue growth. For some children who must be maintained on Dilantin, excessive gum tissue may have to be removed surgically. The growth of gum tissue alone is *not* sufficient reason to switch to other drugs. If the condition leads to emotional problems, disfiguration of the teeth, or related disorders, alternative agents may have to be sought out.

Hirsutism, or excessive growth of body hair, occurs in about 5% of the children treated with Dilantin. Change is most pronounced in arm and leg hair, but the face and trunk may also be affected. The reaction is irreversible, that is, even if medication is stopped the increased hair growth will remain. For cosmetic reasons this may be a problem for teenage girls.

Measlelike rashes are common with Dilantin, beginning within the first 2 weeks of treatment. Such rashes are *not* dose-related, and they clear up when medication is withdrawn.

Another skin reaction that has received attention recently is *coarse facies*, a thickening of the skin of the mouth, nose, and forehead (Falconer & Davidson, 1973). Reports of the prevalence of coarse facies range from 20 to 30% for mentally retarded persons receiving Dilantin in residential facilities (Herberg, 1977; Lefebvre et al., 1972).

The primary gastrointestinal side effect of Dilantin is constipation, which is often encountered in long-term treatment.

The most common side effect of Mesantoin is drowsiness. Other untoward reactions are the same as those for Dilantin intoxication; however, they occur less often for Mesantoin. Rashes are also reported with this medication.

Peganone is not a very powerful antiepileptic and is relatively free of side effects. Untoward reactions that have been reported include rashes, ataxia, diplopia, anorexia, nausea, drowsiness, headache, and dizziness.

Succinimides and Oxazolidinediones

The succinimides are used primarily in the management of absence seizures and consist of three drugs: Zarontin, Celontin (methsuximide), and Milontin (phensuximide). Possible gastrointestinal side effects of Zarontin include abdominal pain, nausea, vomiting, anorexia (loss of appetite), and hiccups. Other reported side effects are drowsiness, headaches, dizziness, and behavioral disturbance. The side effects associated with Celontin and Milontin are similar to those of Zarontin. However, Celontin and Milontin are more likely to produce drowsiness.

The oxazolidinediones (Tridione and Paradione) are also antiabsence agents. *Photophobia*, an aversion to bright light because it is irritating, is the most common side effect of Tridione. Other side effects include headache, diplopia, irritability, drowsiness, rash, nausea, abdominal pain, and hiccups. The untoward reactions associated with Paradione (paramethadione) are similar to those of Tridione.

Other Drugs

Although there was much concern initially about the side effects of Tegretol, Livingston (1978a) commented that after "12 years' experience with the use of carbamazepine in over 1,000 epileptic patients. . . we classify it to be a relatively safe anticonvulsant drug" (p. 306). In one study of 255 epileptic patients treated with Tegretol, 11% became drowsy and 2% exhibited ataxia (Livingston et al., 1974). Either patients developed a tolerance for the drowsiness or the dosage was reduced. In all cases, ataxia responded to dosage reduction. Other reported side effects include nausea, anorexia, and visual disturbances, which appear to be dose-related (see also following section on bone and liver disturbances). One of the major advantages of Tegretol is that it does not appear to impair cognition.

Side effects are frequently reported for Clonopin but rarely are they life threatening (Medical Letter, 1976). Severe drowsiness occurs in nearly half of the individuals treated with Clonopin, ataxia in about a third, and a quarter exhibit behavioral disturbance (aggressivity, irritability, hyperactivity, and agitation). Other side effects include nystagmus, slurred speech, and dysarthria. "Since some patients with the types of seizures (myoclonic and akinetic) for which clonazepam is recommended are severely mentally retarded, the adverse effects of the drug on the patient's ability to perform personal tasks, walk, or communicate may outweigh the benefit of controlling seizures" (p. 19).

The side effects of Depakene are generally considered to be mild and typically abate following dosage reduction (Herranz et al., 1982; Schmidt, 1984). In children the most common adverse reactions are weight gain, drowsiness, gastrointestinal complaints, and hair loss. Gastrointestinal symptoms (loss of appetite, nausea, abdominal pain, and vomiting) have been reduced dramatically with the availability of an enteric-coated preparation (Depakote). Other side effects include tremor, mental confusion, irritability, aggressiveness, and sleep disturbance. Reports of side effects pur portedly due to Depakene are much higher for children who are receiving multiple-drug therapy, and this is probably due to the fact that Depakene inhibits the biotransformation of some antiepileptic drugs (see Drug Interactions). Although Depakene is often recommended as a drug "of first choice," there has been some concern expressed in recent years that statements about the drug's safety should be qualified (e.g., Isom, 1984). There are, for example, a number of reported deaths from Depakene as a consequence of liver damage (see Jeavons, 1984). It is believed that in rare patients (the risk is estimated to be 1 in 20,000) the drug is converted by the liver into toxic metabolites. When this reaction does occur, it typically happens within the first 6 months of treatment. Liver function tests during this period are recommended by many clinicians. Jeavons (1984) concluded his review of this topic by stating that "the best method of avoiding a fatal outcome is clinical monitoring, seeing the patients regularly for the first 6 months, and withdrawing the drug immediately when clinical symptoms of drowsiness, lethargy, vomiting, anorexia, nausea, malaise, oedema, or a clear change in seizure pattern occur'' (p. S53). Young patients receiving multiple drug therapy are at the greatest risk. Another serious but fortunately rare side effect of Depakene is pancreatitis (see Wyllie et al., 1984). Treatment should be discontinued in patients with symptomatic pancreatic disease. Children who experience severe abdominal pain and vomiting on Depakene should undergo blood level monitoring (serum amylase levels) of pancreatic function.

No attempt will be made to discuss the remaining agents with antiepileptic properties in the ''other drugs'' category (see Table 2–1). The interested reader is referred to more comprehensive discussions of pharmacotherapy for seizure disorders (Gilman et al., 1980; Livingston, 1972; Niedermeyer, 1974; Stores, 1978; Woodbury et al., 1982).

Blood, Liver, and Other Disturbances

Certain antiepileptic drugs have an adverse effect upon blood, liver, and kidney functions (Livingston, 1972; Reynolds, 1975). These agents must be monitored closely through both physical examinations and laboratory tests (Livingston, 1978b).

Drugs known to produce blood disturbances in some individuals are Zarontin, Mesantoin, Paradione, Phenurone (phenacemide), and Tridione. While considerable attention is given to blood diseases as a possible side effect of Tegretol, as previously noted, the drug is now considered to be quite safe and serious blood disorders rare. Guidelines for treatment include blood and platelet counts prior to treatment and complete blood counts every 2 weeks for the first 2 months of therapy (see Hart & Easton, 1982). If blood tests are normal, blood counts should then be made every 3 months or upon the occurrence of symptoms of bone marrow suppression. Patients or their parents should be made aware of *possible* signs of blood disease such as fever, sore throat, ulcers in the mouth, easy bruising, *petechial* (small, round, purplish red dot on the surface of the skin) or *purpuric* (purplish or brownish red discoloration beneath the skin) hemorrhage, nosebleed, pale appearance, and undue weakness.

Routine laboratory tests of kidney function must also be conducted for Paradione, Phenurone, and Tridione. Liver function tests must be conducted for Depakene, Tegretol, and Phenurone. Signs of possible liver function disturbance include jaundice, dark urine, general malaise, fever, and gastrointestinal upset.

There is evidence that Dilantin, phenobarbital, and Mysoline interfere with the metabolism of *folic acid* in a small percentage of people receiving either one or a combination of these drugs (Livingston, 1972; Reynolds, 1975). Folic acid is needed by the bone marrow to form red blood cells. When this substance is not present in sufficient quantity, the newly formed red blood cells are much larger than normal, poorly formed, and quite fragile. This condition is called *megoblastic anemia*, and it always responds to treatment with folic acid. In some cases, however, folic acid treatment has increased seizure frequency.

Some investigators have reported abnormally low levels of calcium in the blood *(hypocalcemia)* and bone disorders such as *osteomalacia* and *rickets* in people receiving antiepileptic drugs, particularly Dilantin (Livingston, 1978b; Reynolds, 1975). It has been hypothesized that some antiepileptics stimulate (induce) the metabolism of vitamin D. Thus, vitamin D is removed from the body at a greater rate than normal. Vitamin D is important to bone development because it greatly accelerates the absorption of calcium from the gastrointestinal tract. When the body becomes deficient in vitamin D, calcium is absorbed from the bones. If this situation persists over several months, almost all the calcium in the bones will be absorbed. Then the calcium in the extracellular fluid drops to very low levels. This condition is called *rickets* and is characterized by a weakening of the bones, and, in the later stages, *tetany* (muscle spasms).

The prevalence of drug-induced rickets and osteomalacia and the role of antiepileptic medication is controversial. Most reports for these disturbances are in mentally retarded and/or institutionalized people (Livingston, 1978a). Livingston cited a study in progress that failed to show significant differences in blood calcium levels between epileptic patients on medication and a control group not receiving antiepileptic drugs. One patient who did show abnormally low levels of calcium was administered vitamin D. After reviewing the literature, Livingston concluded that for most people with epilepsy, exposure to sunshine during the summer months is a sufficient source of vitamin D. Patients who are at risk "are those who, because of motor difficulties, severe retardation, or institutionalization, are unable to take advantage of sunshine to form . . . vitamin D" (p. 442).

Cognition, Learning, and School Performance

Interest in the behavioral toxicity of antiepileptic drugs and its clinical implications is not new. Lennox (1942), for example, commented that "many physicians in attempting to extinguish seizures only succeed in drowning the finer intellectual processes of their

patients. . . . The intelligent and individualistic use of anticonvulsant drugs should not and does not impair the patient's mind" (cited
by Trimble & Reynolds, 1976, p. 169). Nevertheless, it has been
within only the last decade that this topic has received much scientific attention.

Surprisingly little research has been conducted on the effects of
antiepileptic drugs on learning, cognition, and school performance.
Much of the information that is available appears as side effect
reports in clinical trials or in case studies. Often, data on dosage,
blood level, and rate at which the reaction occurs are omitted. Many
studies are difficult to interpret because patients were on more than
one drug. The following is a brief summary of the results of a few
studies in this area and their implications for school performance.
For more detailed discussions of cognitive side effects see the literature reviews by Livingston (1972), Stores (1975, 1978), Reynolds
(1983), and Trimble (1979, 1981).

As already mentioned, drowsiness is a common side effect of
antiepileptic medication (particularly phenobarbital and Mysoline),
and many epileptic children are considered by their parents and
teachers to be more drowsy than their peers (Gadow, 1982; Pietsch,
1977). Although in some cases drowsiness may be self-induced as a
manipulative device, others are truly sedated and are occasionally
reprimanded by poorly informed school personnel for laziness.
Obviously, a sedated, sleepy child will have greater difficulty performing school activities. If a child does not develop a tolerance for
the drowsiness within a couple of weeks after the onset of treatment,
the physician can lower the dosage, administer a stimulant (Ritalin
or Dexedrine), or substitute another drug for the offending agent
(Livingston, 1972). If the same dosage that controls seizures also
produces sedation, as Livingston pointed out, a difficult risk-to-
benefit decision will have to be made:

> Some patients may be better off leading a normal life between occa-
> sional seizures than living seizure-free in a perpetual state of drug-
> induced drowsiness and confusion. Both the physician and patient
> must decide which is the greater handicap—the drowsiness or the
> recurrence of seizures. (p. 356)

Another side effect of antiepileptic medication (particularly
phenobarbital) that can seriously impair school performance is
drug-induced behavior disorders, usually hyperactivity. Ways in
which the physician can manage this reaction have already been
noted. There is also another type of behavior disturbance that has
not received much attention (Livingston, 1976). Some behaviorally
normal children become profoundly restless, hyperactive, belliger-

ent, and exhibit frequent temper outbursts after their seizures have been controlled by medication, *regardless of the type of drug*. When medication is stopped or the dosage reduced to the point where seizures reappear, the child's behavior returns to normal. In many cases, the behavior disorder is a greater problem than the seizures. Livingston noted that "in such cases it is probably best to allow the child to have an occasional seizure and normal interictal (between seizures) behavior than to be completely seizure free but with uncontrolled behavior" (p. 259)

Dilantin has been known for many years to produce a confusional state sometimes referred to as *Dilantin encephalopathy*. Because this reaction is generally associated with other clear signs of toxicity such as nystagmus and ataxia, it simply becomes recognized as a sign of Dilantin intoxication and was easily corrected with dosage reduction. In recent years it has been shown that Dilantin produces a variety of behavioral and cognitive symptoms at higher therapeutic and toxic blood levels in the absence of more classical signs of toxicity. These adverse effects include intellectual deterioration, depression, psychomotor slowing, impairment of drive, and aggravation of behavior disorders. The overt classic signs of intoxication may be either overlooked or difficult to detect in mentally retarded or physically handicapped people and in young children. Moreover, researchers have also found behavioral toxicity at blood levels well within the therapeutic range, and there is evidence to suggest that long-term treatment with higher therapeutic dosages of Dilantin may be associated with a deterioration of mental ability (e.g., Corbett et al., 1985; see also Trimble, 1981).

There are growing numbers of systematic investigations of the relationship between high doses or toxic levels of antiepileptic drugs and cognitive performance (Stores, 1975). In one study, Dekaban and Lehman (1975) tested 15 epileptic patients on a number of laboratory tests. Each was receiving one or more of the following agents: phenobarbital, Mysoline, or Dilantin. Among the tasks were a vigilance test and a reaction time test (pressing a button when a light flashed on). Both are paced by the experimenter and require sustained attention. Each patient was tested at the beginning of the study and on two more occasions after a 30 to 50% change in dosage. The majority performed best on both the vigilance and the reaction time tests while on the lowest dose of medication. Eight of the patients felt better subjectively on the lower dose, six could not tell the difference between doses, and one felt better on the highest dose. Dekaban and Lehman noted that heavy medication can impair cognitive performance without there being any clear outward signs of intoxication (e.g., ataxia, diplopia, nystagmus).

Mathews and Harley (1975) compared the performance of two groups of epileptic patients on a number of cognitive and perceptual-motor tests. One group had blood levels of antiepileptic medication in the low toxic range, and the other had nontoxic blood levels. All patients were receiving one or more of the following drugs: phenobarbital, Mysoline, or Dilantin. The most marked differences between the two groups were on measures of sustained concentration, attention span, motor coordination, and motor steadiness, with the nontoxic group performing superior to the toxic group.

Memory processes may also be impaired by high therapeutic doses of barbiturates. MacLeod et al. (1978), for example, compared the performance of epileptic patients receiving a medium and high dose of phenobarbital on short- and long-term memory tasks. The short-term memory task consisted of presenting a series of one to six numbers on a visual display. After a brief pause, a probe number was presented. The patient had to indicate by pressing a lever whether the probe number appeared in the previous display. MacLeod et al. found (relative to a control group) that the high therapeutic dose of phenobarbital impaired short-term memory by increasing the time it took for patients to press the lever. There were no dosage differences on the long-term memory task. These results may have implications for school performance because "impairment of short-term memory may critically influence a person's ability to maintain attention, a crucial ability when one is trying to acquire new information" (p. 1104).

For some children, impairment of cognitive performance will be a necessary price that has to be paid for adequate seizure control. However, in certain treatment populations, special efforts must be made to prevent unnecessary overmedication. For example, a strong argument can be made for the necessity to improve existing drug monitoring procedures for mentally retarded epileptic children and adults (see Chapter 3). One of the anticipated consequences of such efforts would be a reduction in the number of mentally retarded individuals made more intellectually impaired by their medication. Preschoolers constitute another group that requires special attention (see Chapter 3). Because development progresses at such a rapid rate during early childhood, parents, teacher, and physician must seriously consider whether drug-induced mental impairment is a reasonable risk for adequate seizure control. It must be reemphasized that the physical (through injury) and psychological consequences of uncontrolled seizures can also contribute to severe adjustment problems.

Unfortunately, there are no standard procedures for assessing possible impairment of cognitive performance by antiepileptic medication (MacLeod et al., 1978). It is imperative, therefore, that school input be an integral part of the drug evaluation procedure, both at the onset of treatment and during alterations in the drug regimen. At the very least, some effort should be made to establish baseline measures (i.e., prior to treatment) of cognition and behavior, particularly in high-risk cases, so adverse reactions can be adequately assessed. It is hoped that future research efforts will provide more information about what to date has been a much neglected topic—the behavioral side effects of antiepileptic drugs.

PATTERN OF TREATMENT

Drug therapy should be initiated as soon as the diagnosis of epilepsy is made (Livingston, 1978a). In general, the longer the seizures go untreated, the more difficult they are to control. It appears as if each seizure makes the person with a seizure disorder more susceptible to subsequent seizures (see Reynolds, 1982). Drug treatment should be initiated not only to control seizures, but also to prevent seizure-related injuries, brain damage resulting from status epilepticus, emotional disorders, and eventual adjustment problems such as the loss of a job, revocation or denial of a driver's license, and undesirability as a marriage partner.

Whether or not medication should be administered after only one seizure of unknown cause is controversial. Livingston (1958) reported a study of 200 children who had only a single epileptic seizure prior to diagnosis. Children were randomly assigned to one of two groups: continuous phenobarbital therapy or no medication. There was a dramatic decrease in subsequent seizures for the drug-treated group compared with children who were not placed on medication. Livingston's (1978a) position on this issue, presumably based in part on the above study, was as follows:

> We assign the diagnosis of epilepsy to patients who have an unquestionable convulsion of undetermined cause, and we continue with this diagnosis unless the seizure later proves to have been a manifestation of some other disorder. Our general policy is to prescribe daily antiepileptic medication for these patients. . . . It is emphasized, however, that a positive diagnosis of major motor (tonic-clonic) epilepsy, for example, should not be made at the time of the initial

"attack" in a person whose episode was not clearly defined by the observer as a true convulsion unless the EEG reveals abnormalities such as are seen in patients with grand mal epilepsy. (p. 301)

Schedule

There is much controversy as to whether Dilantin and phenobarbital should be administered in a single dose once a day or in divided doses throughout the day. After reviewing the literature, Livingston (1978a) concluded that Dilantin and phenobarbital should be administered to both children and adults at least twice daily because divided doses produce a more even blood level during the day. He further stated that if either of these drugs must be given only once a day, appropriate blood level studies should be conducted. Interviews with parents indicate that almost all children with seizure disorders receive medication in divided doses two or three times per day (Gadow, 1977).

Multiple-Drug Therapy

Another characteristic of antiepileptic drug treatment is the use of two or more drugs for seizure control. The prevalence of multiple-drug therapy ranges from 50% in preschool special education children (Gadow, 1977) and 64% in trainable mentally retarded children (Gadow & Kalachnik, 1981), to 71% in epileptic children surveyed by the National Epilepsy League (Pietsch, 1977). The most common drug combinations are Dilantin and a barbiturate (phenobarbital or Mebaral), Dilantin and Mysoline, and Mysoline and phenobarbital (Gadow, 1977; Gadow & Kalachnik, 1981). The benzodiazepines, succinimides, and oxazoladinediones are rarely used singly. Clinicians have questioned the necessity of *all* these drug combinations and point out that multiple-drug therapy can often be avoided by monitoring drug blood levels (Livingston et al., 1976; Reynolds & Shorvon, 1981; Shorvon & Reynolds, 1977). The usefulness of combining more than three different antiepileptics has also been questioned (Livingston, 1972; Wilson, 1969), but it is easy to see how such a situation could develop for a child whose seizures remain uncontrolled. Studies with adult patients show that single-drug therapy is often better for those with intractable epilepsy (Schmidt, 1983).

Dosage

The average dosages for antiepileptic drugs used at the Samuel Livingston Epilepsy Diagnostic and Treatment Center with children

Table 2–3.   Average Dosages of Antiepileptic Drugs for Children 6 Years of Age and Older*

Drug		Starting Dosage		Maximal Dosage	
		Mg	Times/Day	Mg	Times/Day
Atabrine	quinacrine	50	2	100	3
Bromide		320	3	1000	3
Celontin[1]	methsuximide	300	2	600	4
Clonopin[2]	clonazepam				
Depakene[3]	valproic acid				
Dexedrine	dextroamphetamine	2.5	2	7.5	3
Diamox	acetazolamide	250	2	250	4
Dilantin	phenytoin	100	2	100	4
Gemonil	metharbital	100	3	200	3
Mebaral	mephobarbital	100	3	200	3
Mesantoin[1]	mephenytoin	100	3	400	3
Milontin[1]	phensuximide	500	2	1000	4
Mysoline	primidone	250	3	500	4
Paradione	paramethadione	300	2	600	3
Peganone[1]	ethotoin	500	3	1000	4
Phenobarbital		32	4	65	3
Phonurone[1]	phenacemide	500	3	2000	3
Tegretol[4]	carbamazepine	100	2	100	4
		100	3	200	5
Tridione	trimethadione	300	2	600	3
Valium	diazepam	5	5	10	5
Zarontin	ethosuximide	250	3	500	4

Note: From *Comprehensive Management of Epilepsy in Infancy, Childhood and Adolescence* (p. 198) by S. Livingston, 1972, Springfield, IL: Charles C Thomas. Copyright 1972 by Charles C Thomas, Publisher. Adapted by permission.

* This Table includes only the antiepileptic drugs used at the Samuel Livingston Epilepsy Diagnostic and Treatment Center.

[1] The maximal dosages of these drugs exceeds the manufacturers' recommendations.

[2] In the older child, 1 mg daily is prescribed initially and increased by 0.5 mg to 1 mg every 3 or 4 days to a maximum daily dosage of 6 mg.

[3] Therapy is instituted with a dose of 15 mg/kg/day and this dosage is continued for 2 weeks. If necessary, the dose is subsequently increased as indicated by clinical response or signs of toxicity by 5 to 10 mg/kg/day each week to a maximum of 60 mg/kg/day.

[4] Dosages in first row for 6 to 12 year olds, and dosages in second row for children 13 years and older.

over 6 years of age are listed in Table 2–3. (Drug dosages for children 6 years and under are presented in Chapter 3.) It must be emphasized that these are *average* dosages, and that the actual dose of medication necessary to achieve satisfactory seizure control varies considerably from patient to patient. This is due, in part, to large individual differences in the rate of drug metabolism and removal from the body. The same dose of Dilantin, for example, produces a wide range of blood levels in people with epilepsy (Lascelles et al., 1970). Therefore, whereas one person becomes seizure-free on 200 mg per day of Dilantin, another may require 600 mg daily for adequate seizure control.

Parents and other care providers should be aware that the effect of a particular dose of Dilantin or phenobarbital cannot be adequately evaluated until a stable blood level is reached (Livingston, 1978b). When medication is given orally on a daily basis, the drug gradually accumulates in the blood and eventually levels off. This process may take from 1 to 2 weeks for Dilantin and from 3 to 4 weeks for phenobarbital in adults. A stable blood level of phenobarbital is achieved sooner in children than adults (see Table 2–5). It is also recommended that dosage changes should not be made until the blood level of the drug stabilizes.

Drugs of Choice

Because each of the epilepsies responds best to certain drugs, the extent to which individual antiepileptic agents are used is determined, in part, by the prevalence of the different forms of epilepsy. Therefore, the antitonic-clonic drugs would be expected to be used frequently and the antiabsence agents must less often. Surveys of drug use among children treated for seizure disorders reveal such a distribution (see Chapter 3). By far the most commonly used antiepileptic agents are Dilantin, phenobarbital, and Mysoline.

Duration

Followup studies that investigated the termination of medication show that compared with adults, the prognosis is much better for children who have become seizure-free. After reviewing the limited data available about the withdrawal of antiepileptic medication, Holowach et al. (1972) reported the relapse rate for seizures ranged from 21 to 28% in three studies on children and from 40 to 46% in three studies that included primarily adults. In their own study of 148 cases of childhood seizure disorders, they reported the progno-

sis for tonic-clonic epilepsy was more favorable than for other seizure disorders. The highest relapse rates were for children with
Jacksonian seizures (53%), mixed seizures (40%), and complex partial seizures (25%). Only one of the eight children with absence
spells, all of whom received phenobarbital as a prophylactic measure to prevent the development of tonic-clonic epilepsy, had a
relapse. If seizures have an organic cause and the child is mentally
or motorically retarded, the probability of seizure relapse during
drug withdrawal is greatly increased. The prognosis is best for seizures that have an early onset and are quickly controlled compared
with seizures originating during infancy or later childhood, which
are difficult to bring under control. In general, the longer a person is
on medication and seizure-free, the less likely there will be a relapse
after drug therapy is withdrawn. With the exception of absence seizures, the EEG is of limited value in the decision to withdraw drug
therapy.

Another followup study (Todt, 1984) is worthy of special com-
ment owing to its scope (473 children) and apparent level of sophis-
tication. Briefly, the findings were as follows:

1. The risk of epilepsy relapse (i.e., seizures start again) decreases
   dramatically if dosage withdrawal period is protracted (e.g.,
   relapse for 1-month and 12-month reductions were 70% and
   16%, respectively);
2. The risk of epilepsy relapse decreases dramatically the longer the
   seizure-free period prior to drug withdrawal (e.g., relapse for 1-
   year and 4-year seizure-free periods were 56% and 22%, respectively);
3. For patients who relapsed, their regular drug regimen (i.e., prior
   to drug withdrawal) controlled the seizures in 86% of the cases;
4. Reinstating medication after the first relapse seizure may not be
   necessary;
5. EEG abnormality prior to withdrawal was associated with higher
   relapse rates;
6. The longer the seizure disorder lasts (i.e., the length of time it
   takes to become seizure-free), the greater the risk of relapse;
7. Children who had at least one seizure that lasted 15 minutes or
   longer were at greater risk for relapse; and
8. The discontinuation of medication either during adolescence or
   prior to the onset of adolescence does not appear to be associated
   with greater risk of relapse.

A general rule for the discontinuation of medication for seizure
disorders is to wait at least 4 years after the last seizure before con-

sidering the termination of medication (Livingston, 1972, 1978b). An additional 1 to 4 years may be required for dosage reduction and gradual drug withdrawal, depending upon the dosage of medication that ultimately controlled the seizures and severity of seizures prior to treatment. Sudden discontinuation of medication may precipitate seizures and possibly tonic-clonic status. Occasionally, it is more difficult to control a recurrence of seizures after a sudden withdrawal of medication with the same regimen that was previously effective. If the seizure-free period overlaps the onset of puberty, it may be judicious to continue medication throughout adolescence. This is particularly relevant for females. When the first seizure occurs in late adolescence or early adulthood, it is quite likely that medication will have to be continued throughout the person's lifetime. If seizures occur during the period when the dosage of medication is being reduced, continuous lifetime treatment also is very probable.

ANTIEPILEPTIC DRUG THERAPY DURING PREGNANCY

The reader may wonder why the topic of antiepileptic drug effects on the developing embryo and fetus is included in a book about children and adolescents. There are at least two good reasons for so doing. One, many young females will continue to take medication into adulthood. Two, there is an ever-increasing rate of teenage pregnancies, and there is no reason to believe that adolescents with seizure disorders will be excluded from this social phenomenon.

It has been estimated that from 1 to 8% of all pregnant women have epilepsy (Bossi, 1983), and in most cases the mother has to take medication to protect her and often her unborn child (i.e., a severe seizure that caused the mother to fall or convulse could injure the fetus). Anyone in this situation is obviously going to be concerned about the possible adverse effects of medication. Unfortunately, at the present time, there is no clear-cut answer to the question of whether or not antiepileptic drugs lead to either major or minor birth defects (Bossi, 1983; Philbert & Dam, 1982). Although it is true that untreated (off medication) epileptic mothers are less likely to have children with birth defects than treated (on medication) women, it is not known exactly whether it is the medication, something about the mother (e.g., her genetic background), or both that cause the problem. Nevertheless, there is an increased risk for women who take medication during pregnancy. Before becoming alarmed by this statement, *very careful* consideration should be given to the actual figures reported. Bossi (1983), for example, evaluated the results of 22 retrospective and 9 prospective studies and concluded that the risk of major birth defects for epileptic women was 1¼ to 2 times as great as the risk for nonepileptic women. Fortunately, the prevalence of major congenital malformations is quite low to begin with. As can be seen in Table 2–4, the chance of having a child with a major congenital malformation or malformations is approximately 3 in 100 for both nonepileptic and untreated epileptic mothers. The risk of birth defects is approximately twice as great for those taking medication. Although nearly all types of major congenital malformations have been observed, the most common are heart defects, cleft lip and/or cleft palate, distal limb hypoplasia (incomplete development of hands or feet), clubfoot, and hip dislocation. The results of these studies should not be interpreted to mean that they prove antiepileptic drugs are *teratogenic* (cause birth defects), because women who must take medication probably differ in many important ways from epileptic mothers who stop taking antiepileptic medication during pregnancy (or stopped before they ever became pregnant). Two additional points should also be made in regard to risk factors. First, there is also a greater prevalence of major congenital malformations in offspring of epileptic fathers on medication compared with epileptic fathers who do not take antiepileptic drugs (Meyer, 1973). Second, the search for variables that would predict which mothers are at greatest risk has, for the most, been unsuccessful (see Bossi, 1983).

There are also a variety of more minor defects, sometimes referred to as *minor dysmorphic features*, involving the face, fingers, and toes. They include such features as *ocular hypertelorism* (wide-spaced eyes); inner *epicanthal folds* (a fold of skin on each side of the nose that covers the inside corner of the eye); eye slants; *ptosis* (drooping) of the eyelids; strabismus; flat nasal bridge; low-set, abnormally formed ears; anomalies of the mouth and teeth; and *hypoplasia* of the nails and distal phalanges (incomplete development of finger nails and finger tips). Some of these same features are associated with Down syndrome, fetal alcohol syndrome, and a variety of childhood learning and behavior disorders. These minor defects may occur individually or in combination and are often associated with prenatal and postnatal growth deficiency (i.e., below-average birth weight, small head circumference). The exact prevalence of these minor congenital malformations in children born to women taking antiepileptic medication is not known, but reported rates vary from 6% to 46% (see Andermann et al., 1982; Bossi, 1983). Caregivers should note that these minor dysmorphic

Table 2-4.   Prevalence of Major Congenital Malformations*

Type of Study	Percent Malformed	Number of Studies
1. Epileptic (on and off medication)	5.3	18
versus		
Nonepileptic	3.0	
2. Epileptic (on medication)	7.0	14
versus		
Nonepileptic	4.0	
3. Epileptic (on medication)	8.9	20
versus		
Epileptic (off medication)	3.0	
4. Epileptic (off medication)	2.2	7
versus		
Nonepileptic	3.0	

Note: From "Fetal Effects of Anticonvulsants" by L. Bossi, 1983, in *Antiepileptic Drug Therapy in Pediatrics* (p. 42) by P. L. Morselli, C. E. Pippenger, & J. K. Penry (Eds.). New York: Raven. Copyright 1983 by Raven Press Books, Ltd. Adapted by permission.
*Total number of studies equals 22 retrospective and nine prospective.

features generally do not create problems for children and are fairly common in the general population.

At the present time it is not known if certain malformations are associated with specific drugs or whether or not some antiepileptic drugs are more teratogenic than others. It was once suggested that Dilantin produces its own pattern of cogenital malformations, variously called the *phenytoin syndrome* or *fetal hydantoin syndrome* (Hanson & Smith, 1975), but this notion has since been rejected (e.g., Shapiro et al., 1976).

ANTIEPILEPTIC BLOOD LEVELS

The development of procedures for analyzing the amount of antiepileptic medication in the blood has had a marked effect on the ability to monitor certain aspects of treatment. Although there is quite a bit of variation from child to child as to the amount of drug in the blood necessary for seizure control, there is a good relationship between blood level and signs of intoxication. For example, Jutt (1974) reported that blood levels from 10 to 40 μg/ml are considered in the effective treatment range for phenobarbital. Generally speaking, blood levels below 10 μg/ml are not effective in seizure control, and levels above 40 μg/ml produce adverse reactions. Similar guidelines are available for Dilantin and other antiepileptic drugs (see Table 2–5). Because there is considerable individual variability among children with regard to the pharmacokinetics of antiepileptic drugs, the figures in this table should be considered as being only estimates and used only as general guidelines to clinical management. It goes without saying that blood level information must be considered when making treatment recommendations for it to be really useful (see Beardsley et al., 1983).

There are several situations in which determining the amount of drug in the blood can be quite helpful (Livingston, 1978b). Perhaps the most important is when it is necessary to see if the child is actually taking medication as prescribed. If there is an increase in seizure frequency, a blood level analysis can help determine whether the drug is not controlling the seizures or the child is not taking (swallowing) the medication. If medication was administered as prescribed, a low blood level would indicate that the dosage should be increased. A second indication for monitoring blood level is when signs of intoxication appear at low doses and precise adjustments have to be made. A third situation is identifying which agent is producing intoxication in a multiple-drug regimen. Blood analysis can determine whether one drug is raising or lowering the blood level of another drug. A final indication for using blood monitoring procedures is in the treatment of children who cannot verbally report how the drug is affecting them (e.g., severely mentally retarded individuals) or who exhibit behaviors similar to intoxication (e.g., young children learning to walk may appear ataxic).

DRUG INTERACTIONS

Antiepileptic drugs may interact with one another, with psychotropic drugs, or with a variety of other medicines. When the extent of multiple-drug therapy for epilepsy and the widespread use of non-prescription medicines are considered, it would not be unusual to occasionally encounter such reactions in children receiving antiepileptic medication. On a pharmacokinetic level, many interactions involving antiepileptic drugs can be explained in terms of three processes, plasma protein binding displacement, microsomal enzyme induction, and inhibition of drug metabolism (see Chapter 1). Detailed discussions of drug interactions involving antiepileptic medication have been prepared by Kutt (1984), Levy et al. (1983), Richens (1975), and Woodbury et al. (1982).

Table 2-5. Pharmacologic Properties of Antiepileptic Drugs in Children

Drug	Usual dose (mg/kg/day)	Serum concentration (μg/ml)	Half-life (hours)	Time to steady state (days)	Protein bound (%)
Clonopin (clonazepam)	0.05–0.2	20–80 (ng/ml)	20–40	4–12	< 50
Depakene (valproic acid)	15–60	50–100	6–18	30–75 (hours)	90
Dilantin (phenytoin)	5–10	10–20	12–22	2–5	90
Mysoline (primidone)	12–25	5–10	12	20–30 (hours)	< 50
phenobarbital	4–6	15–40	40–70	8–15	40
Tegretol (carbamazepine)	10–15	6–12	9–19	2–4	70
Zarontin (ethosuximide)	15–35	40–100	30–50	6–12	0

Depakene, Dilantin, Tegretol, and Valium exhibit extensive plasma protein binding (see Table 2–5). When another drug (X) displaces bound antiepileptic drug (Y) molecules, this produces an increase in the level of unbound drug Y molecules. An increase in the latter ultimately leads to an increase in drug clearance (excretion), which in turn results in lower blood concentration of the displaced drug (Y). An example of such an interaction is when salicylate (e.g., aspirin) displaces Dilantin from plasma protein binding sites (Fraser et al., 1980). Fortunately, this particular interaction appears to be clinically benign (see Kutt, 1982).

Several antiepileptic drugs (e.g., Dilantin, Mysoline, phenobarbital, and Tegretol) are microsomal enzyme inducers. In other words, they stimulate a greater production of microsomal enzymes within the liver, which in turn leads to a faster rate of drug metabolism. An example may help to clarify this relationship. Dilantin is a powerful inducer of Tegretol biotransformation (i.e., Dilantin causes the body to produce a greater quantity of enzymes that break down Tegretol). When a person who is receiving Tegretol is given Dilantin to help improve seizure control, the blood level of Tegretol may drop dramatically (see Kutt, 1984).

Another type of interaction occurs when one drug slows down the biotransformation of a second drug. Many drugs, for example, can inhibit the metabolism of Dilantin (Kutt, 1974). When the rate at which Dilantin is broken down into inactive metabolites is slowed down, the level of active drug molecules in the blood increases. This could result in greater seizure control if the child is still having attacks, Dilantin intoxication, or both. It is noteworthy that if the blood level of Dilantin gets too high, the drug may provoke a seizure or *increase* the frequency of attacks (Levy & Fenichel, 1965).

Interactions for commonly prescribed antiepileptic drugs are presented in Table 2–6. To use this table properly, the reader must proceed from left to right. For example, blood levels of phenobarbital (the fourth drug listed) may increase when Depakene is added to the treatment regimen. The mechanism for this phenomenon is the inhibition of drug metabolism. This is clinically important because, as was discussed in Chapter 1, inhibition typically occurs fairly soon (within hours) after the drug combination is initiated. Caregivers should, therefore, be prepared for this situation. Decreases in antiepileptic drug blood levels could be due to plasma protein displacement, microsomal enzyme induction, or both. As for the drugs in Table 2–6, induction is generally the associated process. Unlike inhibition, induction reactions generally develop more gradually over time (weeks to months).

Table 2–6. Possible Changes in Blood Concentrations Consequent to Multiple–Antiepileptic Drug Therapy

Affected Agent	DEP	DIL	MYS	PHE	TEG	ZAR
Depakene (DEP)	NA	—		—	—	
Dilantin (DIL)	—	NA		±		
Mysoline (MYS)	+	—	NA			
phenobarbital (PHE)	+			NA		
Tegretol (TEG)		—	—	—	NA	—
Zarontin (ZAR)	+					NA

Note: Increase in blood level = plus (+); decrease in blood level = minus (−); and NA = not applicable.

Although Table 2–6 presents a convenient overview of potential drug interactions, some additional comments are warranted. First, phenobarbital may affect Dilantin blood levels through both induction and inhibition. The net result appears to be that Dilantin concentrations are relatively unaffected (Windorfer & Sauer, 1977). Second, interactions between Mysoline and other drugs are complicated by the fact that the liver converts Mysoline into two active metabolites, phenobarbital and phenylethylmalonamide (PEMA) (Callaghan et al., 1977; Finchman & Schottelius, 1982). Third, several antiepileptic drugs enhance Depakene biotransformation so that effective blood levels may be difficult to achieve in the presence of other medication. It has been recommended by some, therefore, that Depakene should be used alone (Henriksen & Johannessen, 1980). If used with Dilantin or Tegretol, Depakene levels should be monitored when either drug is added to or withdrawn from the treatment regimen. Fourth, Table 2–6 lists only those interactions that are fairly well established and are somewhat probable. The clinical literature records many more possibilities, but they are either inconsistently documented or rare.

The two most common types of antiepileptic drug interactions that have clinical implications are between (a) Depakene and phenobarbital or Depakene and Dilantin, and (b) Tegretol and other antiepileptic drugs (Levy et al., 1983). The first interaction occurs when Depakene is added to the treatment regimen of a child who is already receiving phenobarbital, Dilantin, or both. In the case of phenobarbital, Depakene inhibits the metabolism of this drug, which may result in an increase in phenobarbital blood concentrations to a toxic level. Possible adverse effects of this drug interaction may be masked by an apparent increase in alertness due to a reduction in seizure frequency. It is recommended, therefore, that the level of phenobarbital concentration be routinely assessed whenever Depakene is added to the treatment regimen. In the case of a child receiving Dilantin, the addition of Depakene may cause Dilantin blood levels to either increase or decrease (decrease is more common) within days, after which there is a return to previous levels over the course of several days or weeks. In some cases, the recovery may take longer or the prior blood level is not attained.

The second most common type of interaction with antiepileptic drugs that requires clinical intervention involves Tegretol. The blood level of this drug generally decreases when used in combination with other antiepileptic agents. Blood levels of Tegretol should be routinely monitored, and an increase in the dosage of Tegretol should be anticipated whenever a new antiepileptic drug is added to a previously stable Tegretol-only drug regimen.

The way in which drug interactions are managed probably varies with the clinician. Shorvon and Reynolds (1977) argued that much unnecessary multiple-drug therapy might be the result of one drug simply elevating another drug to effective levels in the blood. If this were the case, the best thing to do would be to increase the dosage of the effective drug and withdraw the medication that caused the interaction. Unfortunately, things are not always that simple. Both drugs may be required for treatment if one really is not completely effective or if the drugs are being used to control two different types of disorders. In such cases, the dosage of one medication may have to be raised or lowered depending upon the situation. The child and family may be so alarmed by the effects of the drug interaction that the parents terminate the most recently added (presumably offending) agent. It must be emphasized that although antiepileptic drug interactions are possible, they only affect a *small* percentage of patients who receive multiple drugs in such a way that dosage reduction or withdrawal of medication must be employed.

EPILEPSY FOUNDATION OF AMERICA

The Epilepsy Foundation of America (EFA) is a major national agency for people with epilepsy sponsoring a wide variety of programs and activities. The EFA provides information on epilepsy and its consequences to any person or group requesting it. Areas include:

1. Information on epilepsy for the patient, family, and friends.
2. Educational materials to individuals and groups dealing with people with seizure disorders.
3. Information on employment, including vocational rehabilitation and training, rights, hiring and insurance regulations, special programs, and the particular employment needs of some people with epilepsy whose seizures are not fully controlled.
4. Specific information on the rights of persons with epilepsy as guaranteed by federal and state statutes.
5. Housing information (mostly about discrimination and alternative living arrangements, such as group homes).
6. Transportation information, including federal and state driving regulations.
7. Health services information, including prevention, diagnosis, treatment, rehabilitation, and maintenance.
8. Information on economic, social, and psychological services, such as disability benefits and supplemental security income, recreational services, and individual and group counseling programs as they might apply to persons with epilepsy and their families.
9. Information on the latest research into the causes, treatment, and prevention of seizures.
10. Information on federal and state programs that affect people with epilepsy.
11. Research grants and fellowships for professionals.
12. Information for teachers and other school personnel provided through individual "School Alert" kits.

Antiepileptic drugs can be very expensive. In order to alleviate the burden placed upon families by the cost of these drugs, the EFA has for years offered a low-cost pharmacy service as a benefit of membership in EFA. For more information please contact the EFA at the following address:

Epilepsy Foundation of America
4351 Garden City Dr.
Landover, MD 20785
(301) 459–3700

SUGGESTED READINGS

Baird, H. W. (1972). *The child with convulsions: A guide for parents, teachers, counselors, and medical personnel.* New York: Grune & Stratton, 1972. (C, P, S)

Dreifuss, F. E. (1983). *Pediatric epileptology.* Littleton, MA: John Wright•PSG. (C)

Gadow, K. D. (1982). School involvement in the treatment of seizure disorders. *Epilepsia, 23,* 215–224. (S)

Kutt, H. (1984). Interactions between anticonvulsants and other commonly prescribed drugs. *Epilepsia, 25* (Suppl. 2), S118–S131. (C)

Livingston, S. (1972). *Comprehensive management of epilepsy in infancy, childhood and adolescence.* Springfield, IL: Charles C Thomas. (C)

Livingston, S. (1977). Psychosocial aspects of epilepsy. *Journal of Clinical Child Psychology, 6,* 6–10. (C, S)

Livingston, S. (1978a). Medical treatment of epilepsy: Part I. *Southern Medical Journal, 71,* 298–310. (C)

Livingston, S. (1978b). Medical treatment of epilepsy: Part II. *Southern Medical Journal, 71,* 432–447. (C)

Morselli, P. L., Pippenger, C. E., & Penry, J. K. (Eds.). (1983). *Antiepileptic drug therapy in pediatrics.* New York: Raven. (C)

Mostofsky, D. I., & Balaschak, B. A. (1977). Psychobiological control of seizures. *Psychological Bulletin, 84,* 723–750. (C)

Philbert, A., & Dam, M. (1982). The epileptic mother and her child. *Epilepsia, 23,* 85–99. (C)

Reynolds, E. H. (1983). Mental effects of antiepileptic medication: A review. *Epilepsia, 24* (Suppl. 2), S85–S95. (C)

Stores, G. (1978). Antiepileptics (anticonvulsants). In J. S. Werry (Ed.), *Pediatric psychopharmacology: The use of behavior modifying drugs in children* (pp. 274–315). New York: Brunner/Mazel. (C)

Svoboda, W. B. (1979). *Learning about epilepsy.* Baltimore: University Park Press. (C, P, S)

Woodbury, D. M., Penry, J. K., & Pippenger, C. E. (Eds.). (1982). *Antiepileptic drugs* (2nd ed.). New York: Raven. (C)

REFERENCES

Aicardi, J., & Chevrie, J. J. (1970). Convulsive status epilepticus in infants and children: A study of 239 cases. *Epilepsia, 11,* 187–197.

Ajmone Marsan, C., & Zivin, L. S. (1970). Factors related to the occurrence of typical paroxysmal abnormalities in the EEG records of epileptic patients. *Epilepsia, 11,* 361–381.

Andermann, E., Dansky, L., Andermann, F., Loughnan, P. H., & Gibbons, J. (1982). Minor congenital malformations and dermatoglyphic alterations in the offspring of epileptic women: A clinical investigation of the teratogenic effects of anticonvulsant medication. In D. Janz, L. Bossi, M. Dam, H. Helge, A. Richens, & D. Schmidt (Eds.), *Epilepsy, pregnancy and the child* (pp. 235–249). New York: Raven.

Asconapé, J., & Penry, J. K. (1984). Some clinical and EEG aspects of benign juvenile myoclonic epilepsy. *Epilepsia, 25,* 108–114.

Beardsley, R. S., Freeman, J. M., & Appel, F. A. (1983). Anticonvulsant serum levels are useful only if the physician appropriately uses them: An assessment of the impact of providing serum level data to physicians. *Epilepsia, 24,* 330–335.

Bossi, L. (1984). Fetal effects of anticonvulsants. In P. L. Morselli, C. E. Pippenger, & J. K. Penry (Eds.), *Antiepileptic drug therapy in pediatrics* (pp. 37–64). New York: Raven.

Callaghan, N., Feely, M., Duggan, F., O'Callaghan, M., & Seldrup, S. (1977). The effect of anticonvulsant drugs which induce liver microsomal enzymes on derived and ingested phenobarbitone levels. *Acta Neurologica Scandinavica, 56*, 1–6.

Commission on Classification and Terminology of the International League Against Epilepsy. (1981). Proposal for revised clinical and electroenchaphalographic classification of epileptic seizures. *Epilepsia, 22*, 480–501.

Cooper, I. S., Amin, I., Riklan, M., Waltz, J. M., & Poon, T. P. (1976). Chronic cerebellar stimulation in epilepsy. *Archives of Neurology, 33*, 559–570.

Corbett, J. A., Trimble, M. R., & Nichol, T. C. (1985). Behavioral and cognitive impairments in children with epilepsy: The long-term effects of anticonvulsant therapy. *Journal of the American Academy of Child Psychiatry, 24*, 17–23.

Currier, R. D., Kooi, K. A., & Saidman, L. J. (1963). Prognosis of "pure" petit mal: A follow-up study. *Neurology, 13*, 959–967.

Cutts, K. K., & Jasper, H. H. (1939). The effect of benzedrine sulphate and phenobarbital on behavior problem children with abnormal electroencephalograms. *Archives of Neurology and Psychiatry, 41*, 1138–1139.

Dekaban, A. S., & Lehman, E. J. B. (1975). Effects of different dosages of anticonvulsant drugs on mental performance in patients with chronic epilepsy. *Acta Neurologica Scandinavica, 52*, 319–330.

DeVivo, D. C. (1983). Myoclonic seizures. In P. L. Morselli, C. E. Pippenger, & J. K. Penry (Eds.), *Antiepileptic drug therapy in pediatrics* (pp. 137–143). New York: Raven.

Dreifuss, F. E. (1983a). *Pediatric epileptology*. Littleton, MA: John Wright•PSG.

Dreifuss, F. E. (1983b). Generalized tonic-clonic seizures. In P. L. Morselli, C. E. Pippenger, & J. K. Penry (Eds.), *Antiepileptic drug therapy in pediatrics* (pp. 145–151). New York: Raven.

Epilepsy Foundation of America. (1975). *Basic statistics on the epilepsies*. Philadelphia: F. A. Davis.

Falconer, M. A., & Davidson, S. (1973). Coarse features in epilepsy as a consequence of anticonvulsant therapy. *Lancet, 2*, 1112–1114.

Fazio, C., Manfredi, M., & Piccinelli, A. (1973). Treatment of epileptic seizures with clonazepam. *Archives of Neurology, 32*, 304–307.

Fincham, R. W., & Schottelius, D. D. (1982). Primidone. Interactions with other drugs. In D. M. Woodbury, J. K. Penry, & C. E. Pippenger (Eds.), *Antiepileptic drugs* (2nd ed., pp. 421–429). New York: Raven.

Force, D. (1965). *A descriptive study of the incidence of seizures and teachers' attitudes toward children with epilepsy in the Minneapolis, Minnesota Public Schools*. Minneapolis: Minnesota Epilepsy League.

Fraser, D. G., Ludden, T. M., Evans, R. P., & Sutherland, E. W. (1980). Displacement of phenytoin from plasma binding sites by salicylate. *Clinical Pharmacology and Therapeutics, 27*, 165–169.

Gadow, K. D. (1977). *Psychotropic and antiepileptic drug treatment with children in early childhood special education*. Champaign, IL: Institute for Child Behavior and Development, University of Illinois. (ERIC Document Reproduction Service No. ED 162 294)

Gadow, K. D. (1978, May). *Drug therapy with trainable mentally retarded children in public schools.* Paper presented at the annual meeting of the Council for Exceptional Children, Kansas City, Missouri. (ERIC Document Reproduction Service No. ED 153 398)

Gadow, K. D. (1982). School involvement in the treatment of seizure disorders. *Epilepsia, 23,* 215–224.

Gadow, K. D., & Kalachnik, J. (1981). Prevalence and pattern of drug treatment for behavior and seizure disorders of TMR students. *American Journal of Mental Deficiency, 85,* 588–595.

Gastaut, H. (1970). Clinical and electroencephalographical classification of epileptic seizures. *Epilepsia, 11,* 104–113.

Gilman, A. G., Goodman, L. S., & Gilman, A. (Eds.). (1980). *The pharmacological basis of therapeutics.* (6th ed.). New York: Macmillan.

Gold, A. P. (1974). Psychomotor epilepsy in childhood. *Pediatrics, 53,* 540–542.

Goodyer, I. M. (1985). Epileptic and pseudoepileptic seizures in childhood and adolescence. *Journal of the American Academy of Child Psychiatry, 24,* 3–9.

Gram, L., Wulff, K., Rasmussen, K. E., Flachs, H., Würtz-Jørgensen, A., Sommerbeck, K. W., & Løhren, V. (1977). Valproate sodium: A controlled clinical trial including monitoring of drug blood levels. *Epilepsia, 18,* 141–148.

Hanson, J. W., & Smith, D. W. (1975). The fetal hydantoin syndrome. *Journal of Pediatrics, 87,* 285–290.

Hart, R. G., & Easton, J. D. (1982). Carbamazepine and hematological monitoring. *Annals of Neurology, 11,* 309–312.

Henriksen, D., & Johannessen, S. I. (1980). Clinical observation of sodium valproate in children: An evaluation of therapeutic serum levels. In S. I. Johannessen, P. L. Morselli, C. E. Pippenger, A. Richens, D. Schmidt, & H. Meinardi (Eds.), *Antiepileptic therapy: Advances in drug monitoring* (pp. 253–258). New York: Raven.

Herberg, K. P. (1977). Effects of diphenylhydantoin in 41 epileptics institutionalized since childhood. *Southern Medical Journal, 70,* 19–24.

Herranz, J. L., Armijo, J. A., & Arteaga, R. (1984). Effectiveness and toxicity of phenobarbital, primidone, and sodium valproate in the prevention of febrile convulsions, controlled by plasma levels. *Epilepsia, 25,* 85–95.

Herranz, J. L., Arteaga, R., & Armijo, J. A. (1982). Side effects of sodium valproate in monotherapy controlled by plasma levels: A study in 88 pediatric patients. *Epilepsia, 23,* 203–214.

Holowach, J., Thurston, D. L., & O'Leary, J. (1972). Prognosis in childhood epilepsy: Follow-up study of 148 cases in which therapy has been suspended after prolonged anticonvulsant control. *New England Journal of Medicine, 286,* 169–174.

Huf, R., & Schain, R. J. (1980). Longterm experiences with carbamazepine in children with seizures. *Journal of Pediatrics, 37,* 310–312.

Huttenlocher, P. R., Wilbourn, A. J., & Signore, J. M. (1971). Medium-chain triglycerides as a therapy for intractable childhood epilepsy. *Neurology, 21,* 1097–1103.

Isom, J. B. (1984). On the toxicity of valproic acid. *American Journal of Diseases of Children, 138,* 901–903.

Jeavons, P. M. (1977). Nosological problems of myoclonic epilepsies in childhood and adolescence. *Developmental Medicine and Child Neurology, 19,* 3–8.

Jeavons, P. M. (1984). Non-dose-related side effects of valproate. *Epilepsia, 25* (Suppl. 1), S50–S55.

Jeavons, P. M., & Clark, J. E. (1974). Sodium valproate in treatment of epilepsy. *British Medical Journal, 2,* 584–586.

Kutt, H. (1974). The use of blood levels of antiepileptic drugs in clinical practice. *Pediatrics, 53,* 557–560.

Kutt, H. (1982). Phenytoin interactions with other drugs. In D. M. Woodbury, J. K. Penry, & C. E. Pippenger (Eds.), *Antiepileptic drugs* (2nd ed., pp. 227–240). New York: Raven.

Kutt, H. (1984). Interactions between anticonvulsants and other commonly prescribed drugs. *Epilepsia, 25* (Suppl. 2), S118–S131.

Kutt, H., & Louis, S. (1972). Untoward effects of anticonvulsants. *New England Journal of Medicine, 286,* 1316–1317.

Lascelles, P. T., Kocen, R. S., & Reynolds, E. H. (1970). The distribution of plasma phenytoin levels in epileptic patients. *Journal of Neurology, Neurosurgery and Psychiatry, 33,* 501–505.

Lee, S. I. (1983). Electroencephalography in infantile and childhood epilepsy. In F. E. Dreifuss, *Pediatric epileptology: Classification and management of seizures in the child* (pp. 33–63). Littleton, MA: John Wright•PSG.

Lefebvre, E. B., Haining, R. G., & Labbé, R. F. (1972). Coarse facies, calverial thickening and hyperphosphatasia associated with long-term anticonvulsant therapy. *New England Journal of Medicine, 286,* 1301–1302.

Lennox, W. G. (1942). Brain injury, drugs and environment as causes of mental decay in epilepsy. *American Journal of Psychiatry, 99,* 174–180.

Lennox, W. G. (1945). Treatment of epilepsy. *Medical Clinics of North America, 29,* 1114–1128.

Lennox, W. G. (1960). *Epilepsy and related disorders.* Boston: Little, Brown.

Levy, L. L., & Fenichel, G. M. (1965). Diphenylhydantoin activated seizures. *Neurology, 15,* 716–722.

Levy, R. H., Moreland, T. A., & Farwell, J. R. (1983). Drug interactions in epileptic children. In P. L. Morselli, C. E. Pippenger, & J. K. Penry (Eds.), *Antiepileptic drug therapy in pediatrics* (pp. 75–84). New York: Raven.

Lindsley, D. B., & Henry, C. E. (1941). The effects of drugs on behavior and the electroencephalograms of children with behavior disorders. *Psychosomatic Medicine, 4,* 140–149.

Little, T. M., Girgis, S. S., & Masotti, R. E. (1975). Diphenylhydantoin-induced gingival hyperplasia: Its response to changes in drug dosage. *Developmental Medicine and Child Neurology, 17,* 421–424.

Livingston, H. L., & Livingston, S. (1973). Diphenylhydantoin gingival hyperplasia. *Pediatric Annals, 2,* 81–92.

Livingston, S. (1958). Convulsive disorders in infants and children. In S. Z. Levine (Ed.), *Advances in pediatrics* (Vol. 10). Chicago: The Year Book.

Livingston, S. (1972). *Comprehensive management of epilepsy in infancy, childhood and adolescence.* Springfield, IL: Charles C Thomas.

Livingston, S. (1974). Diagnosis and treatment of childhood myoclonic seizures. *Pediatrics, 53*, 542–548.

Livingston, S. (1976). Behavioral effects of anti-epileptic drugs. *Developmental Medicine and Child Neurology, 18*, 258–259.

Livingston, S. (1977). Psychosocial aspects of epilepsy. *Journal of Clinical Child Psychology, 6*, 6–10.

Livingston, S. (1978a). Medical treatment of epilepsy: Part I. *Southern Medical Journal, 71*, 298–310.

Livingston, S. (1978b). Medical treatment of epilepsy: Part II. *Southern Medical Journal, 71*, 432–447.

Livingston, S., & Pauli, L. L. (1975). Dextroamphetamine for epilepsy. *Journal of the American Medical Association, 233*, 278–279.

Livingston, S., Pauli, L. L., & Berman, W. (1974). Carbamazepine (Tegretol) in epilepsy: Nine year follow-up study with special emphasis on untoward reactions. *Diseases of the Nervous System, 35*, 103–107.

Livingston, S., Pauli, L. L., & Pruce, I. (1976). Letter: One-drug regimens for epilepsy. *Lancet, 1*, 1407–1408.

Livingston, S., Pauli, L. L., & Pruce, I. (1977). Ketogenic diet in the treatment of epilepsy. *Developmental Medicine and Child Neurology, 19*, 833–834.

Livingston, S., Pauli, L. L., & Pruce, I. (1978). No proven relationship of carbamazepine therapy to blood dyscrasias. *Neurology, 28*, 101–102.

Livingston, S., Torres, I., Pauli, L. L., & Rider, R. V. (1965). Petit mal epilepsy: Results of a prolonged follow-up study of 117 patients. *Journal of the American Medical Association, 194*, 227–232.

Lombroso, C. T. (1974). The treatment of status epilepticus. *Pediatrics, 3*, 536–540.

MacLeod, C. M., Dekaban, A. S., & Hunt, E. (1978). Memory impairment in epileptic patients: Selective effects of phenobarbital concentration. *Science, 202*, 1102–1104.

Mathews, C. G., & Harley, J. P. (1975). Cognitive and motor-sensory performances in toxic and nontoxic epileptic subjects. *Neurology, 25*, 184–188.

Medical Letter. (1976). *18*, 18–19.

Meighan, S. S., Queener, L., & Weitman, M. (1976). Prevalence of epilepsy in children of Multnomah County, Oregon. *Epilepsia, 17*, 245–256.

Merritt, H. H., & Putnam, T. J. (1938). Sodium diphenylhydantoinate in the treatment of convulsive disorders. *Journal of the American Medical Association, 111*, 1068–1073.

Meyer, J. G. (1973). The teratological effects of anticonvulsants and the effects on pregnancy and birth. *European Neurology, 10*, 179–190.

Mikkelsen, B., Birket-Smith, E., Brandt, S., Holm, P., Lund, M., Thorn, I., Vestmark, S., & Olsen, P. A. (1976). Clonazepam in the treatment of epilepsy. *Archives of Neurology, 33*, 322–325.

Millichap, J. G. (1972). Drug therapy: Drug treatment of convulsive disorders. *New England Journal of Medicine, 286*, 464–469.

Mostofsky, D. I., & Balaschak, B. A. (1977). Psychobiological control of seizures. *Psychological Bulletin, 84*, 723–750.

Nelson, K. B., & Ellenberg, J. H. (1978). Prognosis in children with febrile seizures. *Pediatrics, 61,* 720–727.

Niedermeyer, E. (1974). *Compendium of the epilepsies.* Springfield, IL: Charles C Thomas.

Pietsch, S. (Ed.). (1977). *The person with epilepsy: Life style, needs, expectations.* Chicago: National Epilepsy League.

Philbert, A., & Dam, M. (1982). The epileptic mother and her child. *Epilepsia, 23,* 85–99.

Putnam, T. J., & Merritt, H. H. (1937). Experimental determination of the anticonvulsant properties of some phenyl derivatives. *Science, 85,* 525–526.

Reynolds, E. H. (1975). Chronic antiepileptic toxicity: A review. *Epilepsia, 16,* 319–352.

Reynolds, E. H. (1982). The pharmacological management of epilepsy associated with psychological disorders. *British Journal of Psychiatry, 141,* 549–557.

Reynolds, E. H. (1983). Mental effects of antiepileptic medication: A review. *Epilepsia, 24* (Suppl. 2), S85–S95.

Reynolds, E. H., & Shorvon, S. D. (1981). Monotherapy or polytherapy for epilepsy? *Epilepsia, 22,* 1–20.

Richens, A. (1975). Drug interactions in epilepsy. *Developmental Medicine and Child Neurology, 17,* 94–95.

Rodin, E. A., Rim, C. S., Kitano, H., Lewis, R., & Rennick, P. M. (1976). A comparison of the effectiveness of primidone versus carbamazepine in epileptic outpatients. *Journal of Nervous and Mental Disease, 163,* 41–46.

Rose, S. W., Penry, J. K., Markush, R. E., Radlof, L. A., & Putnam, P. L. (1973). Prevalence of epilepsy in children. *Epilepsia, 14,* 133–152.

Sato, S. (1983). Generalized seizures: Absence. In F. E. Dreifuss, *Pediatric Epileptology* (pp. 65–91). Littleton, MA: John Wright•PSG.

Sato, S., White, B. G., Penry, J. K., Dreifuss, F. E., Sackellares, J. C., & Kupferberg, H. J. (1982). Valproic acid versus ethosuximide in the treatment of absence seizures. *Neurology, 32,* 157–163.

Schain, R. J. (1983). Carbamazepine and cognitive functioning. In P. L. Morselli, C. E. Pippenger, & J. K. Penry (Eds.), *Antiepileptic drug therapy in pediatrics* (pp. 189–192). New York: Raven.

Schmidt, D. (1983). Reduction of two-drug therapy in intractable epilepsy. *Epilepsia, 24,* 368–376.

Schmidt, D. (1984). Adverse effects of valproate. *Epilepsia, 25* (Suppl. 1), S44–S49.

Shapiro, S., Hartz, S. C., Siskind, V., Mitchell, A. A., Slone, D., Rosenberg, L., Monson, R. R., & Heinonen, O. P. (1976). Anticonvulsants and parental epilepsy in the development of birth defects. *Lancet, 1,* 272–275.

Sherwin, A. L. (1983). Absence seizures. P. L. Morselli, C. E. Pippenger, & J. K. Penry (Eds.), *Antiepileptic drug therapy in pediatrics* (p. 153–161). New York: Raven.

Shorvon, S. D., & Reynolds, E. H. (1977). Unnecessary polypharmacy for epilepsy. *British Medical Journal, 1,* 1635–1637.

Signore, J. M. (1973). Ketogenic diet containing medium-chain triglycerides. *Journal of the American Dietetic Association, 62,* 285–290.

Stores, G. (1975). Behavioral effects of antiepileptic drugs. *Developmental Medicine and Child Neurology, 17,* 647–658.

Stores, G. (1978). Antiepileptics (anticonvulsants). In J. S. Werry (Ed.), *Pediatric psychopharmacology: The use of behavior modifying drugs in children* (pp. 274–315). New York: Brunner/Mazel.

Stores, G. (1985). Clinical and EEG evaluation of seizures and seizure-like disorders. *Journal of the American Academy of Child Psychiatry, 24,* 10–16.

Thorn, I. (1975). A controlled study of prophylactic long term treatment of febrile convulsions with phenobarbital. *Acta Neurologica Scandinavica Supplementum, 60,* 67–73.

Todt, H. (1984). The late prognosis of epilepsy in childhood: Results of a prospective follow-up study. *Epilepsia, 25,* 137–144.

Trauner, D. A. (1985). Medium-chain triglyceride (MCT) diet in intractable seizure disorders. *Neurology, 35,* 237–238.

Trimble, M. (1979). The effect of anticonvulsant drugs on cognitive abilities. *Pharmacology and Therapeutics, 4,* 677–685.

Trimble, M. (1981). Anticonvulsant drugs, behavior, and cognitive abilities. In W. B. Essman & L. Valzelli (Eds.), *Current developments in psychopharmacology* (Vol. 6, pp. 65–91). New York: Spectrum.

Trimble, M. R. & Reynolds, E. H. (1976). Anticonvulsant drugs and mental symptoms: A review. *Psychological Medicine, 6,* 169–178.

Williams, D. T., & Mostofsky, D. I. (1982). Psychogenic seizures in childhood and adolescence. In T. Riley & A. Roy (Eds.), *Pseudoseizures.* Baltimore: Williams & Wilkins.

Wilson, J. (1969). Drug treatment of epilepsy in childhood. *British Medical Journal, 4,* 475–477.

Windorfer, A., & Sauer, W. (1977). Drug interactions during anticonvulsant therapy in childhood: Diphenylhydantoin, primidone, phenobarbital, clonazepam, nitrazepam, carbamazepine and depropylacetate. *Neuropädiatrie, 8,* 29–41.

Wolf, S. M., Carr, A., Davis, D. C., Davidson, S., Dale, E. P., Forsythe, A., Goldenberg, E. D., Hanson, R., Lulejian, G. A., Nelson, M. A., Treitman, P., & Weinstein, A. (1977). The value of phenobarbital in the child who has had a single febrile seizure: A controlled prospective study. *Pediatrics, 59,* 378–385.

Wolf, S. M., & Forsythe, A. (1978). Behavior disturbance, phenobarbital, and febrile seizures. *Pediatrics, 61,* 728–731.

Woodbury, D. M., Penry, J. K., & Pippenger, C. E. (Eds.). (1982). *Antiepileptic drugs* (2nd ed.). New York: Raven.

Wyllie, F., Wyllie, R., Cruse, R. P., Erenberg, G., & Rothner, A. D. (1984). Pancreatitis associated with valproic acid therapy. *American Journal of Diseases of Children, 138,* 912–914.

Zimmerman, F. T., & Burgemeister, B. B. (1958). A new drug for petit mal epilepsy. *Neurology, 8,* 769–775.

Zlutnick, S., Mayville, W. J., & Moffat, S. (1975). Modification of seizure disorders: The interruption of behavioral chains. *Journal of Applied Behavior Analysis, 8,* 1–12.

Chapter **3**

Seizure Disorders: Early Childhood and Mental Retardation

Seizure disorders occur with much greater frequency in children and adolescents who have experienced some type of injury to the brain. Therefore, it is not surprising that surveys of educational and habilitative programs that serve people with severe or profound mental retardation, cerebral palsy, or multiple handicaps report relatively high rates of antiepileptic drug therapy. It also follows that the care providers who staff these programs and facilities encounter epilepsy on a regular basis, a fact that has important implications for professional training. As for the people who are the recipients of these services, the needs and problems created by their seizure disorder, their underlying handicapping conditions, and their medication often interact in ways that create a special set of treatment-related concerns. This chapter addresses these concerns for two populations of school-aged children, the mentally retarded and the young handicapped child.

EARLY CHILDHOOD

Early childhood is one of the peak periods for the development of seizure disorders, particularly the first 2 years of life. The actual percentage of preschool-aged children who are receiving antiepileptic medication is difficult to determine, but the figure is probably between 1/2 and 1%. The drug prevalence rates for special education facilities and programs, however, are much higher. This is due, in part, to the fact that some of the mechanisms that produce various types of handicaps (e.g., brain damage) are associated in some often unexplained way with seizure disorders. For example, children with more severe forms of cerebral palsy and mental retardation often have seizure disorders.

Although most types of seizure disorders occur in young children, a few are found only during early childhood (e.g., neonatal seizures, infantile spasms, and febrile seizures) and others such as absence seizures (petit mal) and certain types of myoclonic epilepsy generally first begin at this time (see Dreifuss, 1983; Livingston, 1972; Morselli et al., 1983). Tonic-clonic (grand mal) seizures are the most common, whereas complex partial (psychomotor) seizures are infrequent. Because each type of seizure disorder and its medical management are described in some detail in Chapter 2, they are not discussed here. Rather, what is presented is a description of patterns of drug use with children in early childhood special education (ECSE) programs and particular aspects of antiepileptic drug use that have special significance for this period of development.

Pattern of Treatment

Most of what is known about the prevalence and pattern of antiepileptic drug use with young children (between 3 and 5 years old) is from two survey studies of ECSE programs (Gadow, 1975, 1977). It was found that 6.6% of the youngsters were taking medication for seizures (Fig. 3–1). Although it was not possible to determine the type of seizure for which each medicine was prescribed, the findings do permit an overview of medication use on a large scale. Table 3–1 lists all reported drugs and the number of children who received each. The data for two groups of preschool-aged children are presented. One group (SD) received medication for a seizure disorder only. The second group (SD-BD) were treated concurrently for both a behavior and a seizure disorder; however, only the antiepileptic drugs are listed. As is clear from Table 3–1, the most commonly prescribed antiepileptic drugs were phenobarbital, Dilantin (phenytoin), Mysoline (primidone), and Valium (diazepam). A few antiepileptic drugs are either underrepresented or not listed because they were either introduced (Clonopin, Depakene) or became more widely used (Tegretol) after these studies were conducted. Tonic-clonic (grand mal) seizures are the most common type of seizure disorder, so it is not surprising that antiepileptic drugs effective for these seizures (e.g., Dilantin, phenobarbital, and Mysoline) are the most widely used. Absence seizures are generally treated with dif-

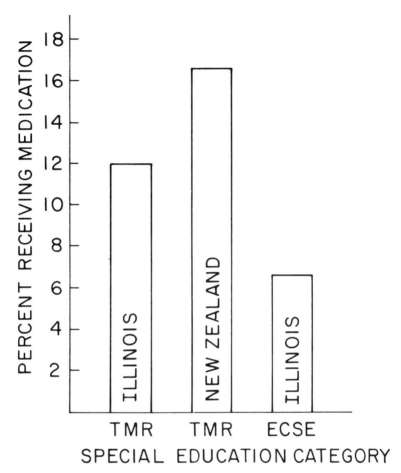

Figure 3–1. Percentage of children in classes for the trainable mentally retarded (TMR) and in early childhood special education (ECSE) receiving medication for a seizure disorder.

ferent medications (e.g., Depakene, Zarontin), but only 6 to 12% of the children with seizure disorders have this type of seizure so these drugs are reported as being used less frequently. It is noteworthy that phenobarbital, a drug that often produces a behavioral side effect that is similar to hyperactivity, was used infrequently with the SD-BD group.

Over one half of the ECSE children treated for a seizure disorder received two or more antiepileptic drugs in combination (Fig. 3–2). Multiple-drug therapy *may* be necessary for several reasons (Livingston, 1972). One, an initial drug may be helpful in reducing the frequency and severity of seizures but yet not completely adequate

Table 3-1. Drugs Prescribed for the Management of Seizure Disorders in Preschool-Aged Children

Generic Name	Trade Name	SD(N = 140)[a]	SD-BD(N = 24)[a]
Phenobarbital		76	2
Phenytoin	Dilantin	59	19
Primidone	Mysoline	19	4
Diazepam	Valium	11	2
Mephobarbital	Mebaral	7	1
Acetazolamide	Diamox	3	0
Carbamazepine	Tegretol	3	0
Metharbital	Gemonil	3	0
Methsuximide	Celontin	3	2
Other		21	2
Total[b]		205	32

Note: From *Psychotropic and Antiepileptic Drug Treatment in Early Childhood Special Education* (p. 24, 27) by K. D. Gadow, 1977, Institute for Child Behavior and Development, University of Illinois at Urbana-Champaign. (ERIC Document Reproduction Service No. ED 162 494)

[a] SD = on medication for seizure disorder; SD-BD = on medication for both behavior and seizure disorder.

[b] Totals are inflated because many children received two or more drugs during the school year.

for total seizure control. Another agent may be added to see if therapeutic response can be improved, and two or three drugs may be necessary if the seizures are particularly frequent or severe. Two, the management of absence seizures may involve an antiabsence drug as well as an antitonic-clonic agent. The latter is prescribed as a prophylactic measure to prevent the development of tonic-clonic seizures. Three, because many children with seizure disorders have more than one kind of seizure (Livingston, 1972), it may be necessary to use different medicines to control the different types of seizures. Although multiple-drug therapy may be necessary to achieve adequate control of seizures in some cases, the efficacy of prescribing more than three has been called into question (Livingston, 1972; Wilson, 1969). At the present time, there is a growing consensus that treatment with one medication is best (see Chapter 2), unless an additional drug is absolutely necessary. The most frequently reported drug combinations for ECSE children were Dilantin and a barbiturate, Dilantin and Mysoline, and Mysoline and phenobarbital. For ECSE children receiving only one medication, phenobarbital was the most frequently reported drug (54%) and Dilantin second (23%). Valium and the succinimides (Zarontin and Celontin) were

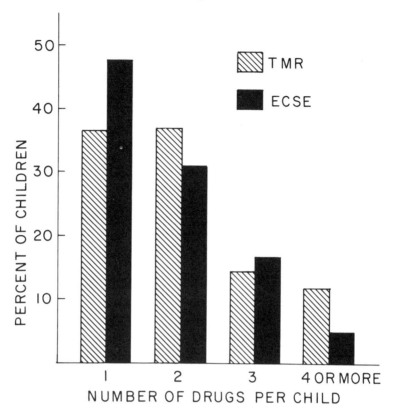

Figure 3–2. Number of drugs administered per child per day. *Note:* From *Psychotropic and Antiepileptic Drug Treatment in Early Childhood Special Education* (p. 32) by K. D. Gadow, 1977, Institute for Child Behavior and Development, University of Illinois at Urbana-Champaign. (ERIC Document Reproduction Service No. 162 494)

always reported as being used in combination with other antiepileptic drugs.

All the parents of ECSE children who were interviewed about the effectiveness of antiepileptic medication said that it helped their child, by reducing either the severity or the frequency of the seizures. However, seizure control was not always complete. Over one third said that their child still experienced seizures, and the frequency varied greatly depending upon the type of seizure and the child. When asked if their child had a seizure within the last 6 months, 57% of the parents responded affirmatively. So while antiepileptic medication is generally very effective, it does not always produce complete seizure control. And, in certain types of seizure disorders that are generally associated with mental retardation, such as infantile spasms or some types of myoclonic epilepsy, medication may be of little benefit at all. In some cases seizures occur as a result of not giving medication in the prescribed manner.

A number of clinicians have expressed concern about antiepileptic drug therapy with preschool-age children (e.g., Cordes, 1973; Dekaban & Lehman, 1975). The primary consideration is that the dosage of medication should not be so high, as it impairs adaptive behavior, which may be very difficult to assess in young handicapped children. Cordes (1973), for example, described a case study of a preschool girl who developed mild mental retardation on antiepileptic medication. Termination of treatment was followed by a marked developmental spurt. About another preschool child receiving multiple drugs for minor motor seizures, a mother commented, "Each time he comes off another pill learning increases and the school has less problems" (Gadow, 1977, p. 46). Cordes (1973) concluded his case study with the following appeal for careful clinical management:

> Children, because of the rapidity, the intricacy, and the vulnerability of their developmental and maturational processes, are exquisitely sensitive to any interference with these processes that. . .once a critical developmental stage has been distorted or delayed, it is not easily recoverable (and) sedative drugs such as phenobarbital (and probably other sedative and tranquilizing drugs as well) are potent interfering agents with these delicate processes. . . .Chronic intoxication in a young child is almost always iatrogenic, usually in an attempt to treat some condition such as a convulsive disorder or possibly a behavioral abnormality. If further cases such as June's can be documented, then perhaps all physicians who deal with preschool children can have a clearer idea of their responsibility, and their need, for the most precise clinical judgment when prescribing any sedative or tranquilizing drug for a young child. (pp. 221–222)

Antiepileptic drugs are generally administered in divided dosages (two or more times a day) to children (Fig. 3–3). The reason for this is that it is believed that divided doses produce more constant or even blood levels than a single daily dose (Svensmark & Buchthal, 1964) and that this leads to better seizure control and fewer side effects. There remains, however, some controversy over these assumptions. As can be seen in Figure 3–3, morning and evening are the most common times for drug administration, with about one half taking medicine at noon.

General dosage guidelines for children under 6 years of age for most antiepileptic drugs available in the United States are presented in Table 3–2. Additional information about these drugs, their use, and associated side effects are presented in Chapter 2.

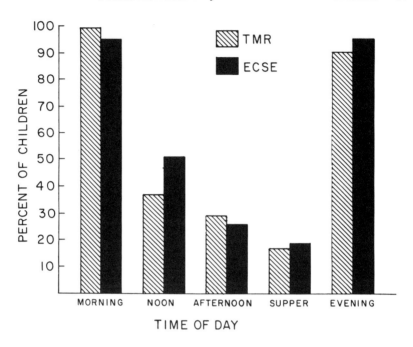

Figure 3-3. Time of day children treated for a seizure disorder received medication. *Note:* From *Psychotropic and Antiepileptic Drug Treatment in Early Childhood Special Education* (p. 36) by K. D. Gadow, 1977, Institute for Child Behavior and Development, University of Illinois at Urbana-Champaign. (ERIC Document Reproduction Service No. 162 494)

MENTAL RETARDATION

Drug treatment for seizure disorders in mentally retarded children, adolescents, and adults is considered a separate topic in this book for several reasons. First, seizure disorders are a common malady in mentally retarded populations. This is particularly true for more severely and profoundly impaired individuals. Second, mental retardation is a common disability in children with certain types of seizures such as infantile spasms and Lennox-Gastaut syndrome. Third, because several different types of disorders are commonly associated with mental retardation, the prevalence of multiple-drug regimens is also greater. And fourth, the way in which social agencies and the general public respond to mentally retarded people may interact in complex ways with decisions about drug treatment. For example, the recent emphasis on deinstitutionalization is bringing many severely and profoundly retarded persons into the mainstream of everyday life through community placements. The feasibility of

Table 3–2. Average Dosages of Antiepileptic Drugs for Children Under 6 Years of Age*

Trade Name	Generic Name	Age (years)	Starting Dosage		Maximal Dosage	
			Mg	Times/Day	Mg	Times/Day
(ACTH and corticosteroids)[1]						
Atabrine	quinacrine	Under 6	50	1	50	3
(Bromide)		Under 3	160	2	320	3
		3 to 6	320	2	640	3
Celontin	methsuximide	Under 6	150	3	300	4
Clonopin[2]	clonazepam					
Depakene[3]	valproic acid					
Dexedrine	dextroamphetamine	Under 6	2.5	1	2.5	3
Diamox	acetazolamide	Under 6	125	3	250	3
Dilantin[4]	phenytoin	Under 2	15	3	30	3
		2 to 4	30	2	50	4
		4 to 6	30	3	100	3
Gemonil	metharbital	Under 6	50	3	100	3
Mebaral	mephobarbital	Under 2	32	3	50	4
		2 to 4	32	4	82	3
		4 to 6	50	4	100	3
Mesantoin	mephenytoin	Under 6	50	3	200	3
Milontin	phensuximide	Under 6	250	2	500	3
Mysoline	primidone	Under 2	25	2	50	4
		2 to 4	50	3	125	4
		4 to 6	125	3	250	4
Paradione	paramethadione	Under 6	150	2	300	3

Peganone	ethotoin	Under 6	250	3	750	4
(phenobarbital)		Under 2	16	3	32	3
		2 to 4	16	4	32	4
		4 to 6	32	3	48	3
Phenurone	phenacemide	Under 6	250	3	1000	3
Tegretol	carbamazepine	Under 6	100	1	100	3
Tridione	trimethadione	Under 6	150	2	300	3
Valium[5]	diazepam					
Zarontin	ethosuximide	Under 6	250	2	250	4

Note: From Comprehensive *Management of Epilepsy in Infancy, Childhood, and Adolescence* (p. 198) by S. Livingston, 1972, Springfield, IL: Charles C Thomas. Copyright 1972 by Charles C Thomas, Publisher. Adapted by permission.

* This Table includes only the antiepileptic drugs used at the Samuel Livingston Epilepsy Diagnostic and Treatment Center.

[1] The patient should receive a daily intramuscular injection of 20 units of corticotropin twice daily for 4 to 6 weeks, depending upon seizure response. If complete control of seizures and normalization of the EEG are obtained, no further therapy is indicated unless there is a recurrence of clinical seizures. If, after 6 weeks of treatment with ACTH, clinical control of seizures is attained but the EEG remains abnormal, steroid therapy (cortisone or prednisone) should be instituted and continued for a prolonged period in an attempt to normalize the EEG. If there is no clinical response to 6 weeks of ACTH therapy, the patient may be given a trial of oral steroid therapy, administered daily for at least 2 months. It is important that oral steroid therapy be discontinued gradually.

[2] Therapy in younger children is initiated with a daily dose of 0.5 mg and increased by increments of 0.25 to 0.5 mg every 3 to 4 days to a maximum daily dosage of 3 mg.

[3] Therapy is instituted with a dose of 15 mg/kg/day and this dosage is continued for 2 weeks. If necessary, the dose is subsequently increased as indicated by clinical response or signs of toxicity by 5 to 10 mg/kg/day each week to a maximum of 60 mg/kg/day.

[4] We only rarely prescribe phenytoin for infants.

[5] Effective dosage of diazepam varies from patient to patient. We start treatment as follows: children under age one, 1 mg every 3 hours for 5 doses daily, and young children, 2 mg every 3 hours for 5 doses daily. The daily dose is increased if necessary, by one dosage per week, depending on clinical response and tolerance to the drug. The appearance of marked drowsiness indicates that the maximal tolerable dosage has been surpassed. The maximal daily dosages we have employed: children under age one, 15 mg, and young children, 30 mg. The package insert states that oral diazepam is contraindicated in children under age 6 months and that intravenous diazepam is contraindicated in infants under 30 days of age.

such placements for some individuals with severe seizure disorders *may* depend upon effective pharmacotherapy.

The prevalence of seizure disorders among moderately to profoundly retarded people is much greater than among the general population. Schain (1975) described the relationship between the two disorders as "linked together epidemiologically, etiologically, clinically and therapeutically." Although seizure disorders do not appear to be more prevalent among borderline and mildly retarded individuals than in the general population (Slater & Cowie, 1971), estimates for severely and profoundly retarded persons in residential facilities are as high as 30% (Jasper et al., 1969).

Largely as a result of lawsuits concerning the mistreatment of mentally retarded people in institutions, a fairly substantial amount of information about how pharmacotherapy is managed in real world situations is now available. Although these data were generally not collected in response to a court order, the lawsuits drew enough attention to this area that a number of scientists became interested in documenting the extent of alleged wrongdoing. Drug treatment practices are described here for three different settings: institutions, community placements, and public schools.

Institutions

Payne et al. (1969) conducted what must certainly be one of the most comprehensive surveys of mentally retarded persons in residential facilities. Twenty-two institutions in the Western United States were asked to provide detailed data on a total of 24,257 residents in 1968. It was found that 26% of all the mentally retarded persons in these institutions were receiving medication for seizure control. Institutions with greater proportions of severely and profoundly mentally retarded residents reported the highest rates of antiepileptic drug therapy.

A survey of an institution in Virginia found that approximately 30% were receiving antiepileptic medication (O'Neill et al., 1977). Patients were grouped according to three categories of seizure control: controlled (no seizures for a year), partially controlled (one to three seizures in any quarter of the year), and uncontrolled (four or more seizures in any quarter of the year). Using these categories, 13% were classified as uncontrolled, 24% as partially controlled, and 63% as controlled.

Some of the most extensive studies of institutions have been conducted by Brad Hill at the University of Minnesota (Hill et al., 1983, 1984). In 1977, he and his colleagues identified 55,438 mentally retarded individuals in public residential facilities (institutions) under the age of 22 years in the United States. Staff interviews concerning a randomly selected sample of children and adolescents revealed that 44% were receiving drug treatment for epilepsy (Hill, 1984). Over three fourths of the institutional sample were severely or profoundly retarded (IQ < 36).

The international picture of antiepileptic drug prescribing is fairly consistent. Although there is obviously some variability, approximately 30% of the residents in institutions in Canada (Tu, 1979), England (Kirman, 1975; Spencer, 1974), New Zealand (Pulman et al., 1979), and the United States (Cohen & Sprague, 1977; O'Neill et al., 1977; Payne et al., 1969; Silva, 1979; Sprague, 1977a) are treated for seizure disorders (Fig. 3–4).

Community Placements

The most extensive studies of antiepileptic drug use in specially licensed community residential facilities (e.g., foster homes, group

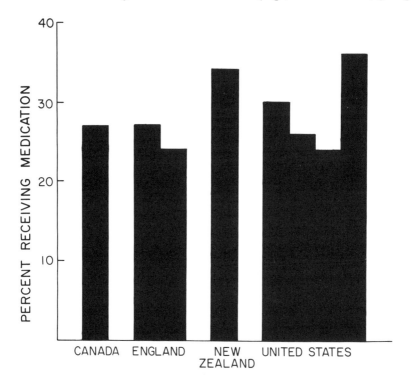

Figure 3–4. Prevalence of drug therapy for seizure disorders in institutions for the mentally retarded as reported in eight surveys.

homes) have also been conducted by Hill and his associates (1983, 1984). In 1977, they identified 35,751 mentally retarded children and adolescents in community residential placements. Staff interviews concerning a randomly selected sample indicated 18% were being treated for a seizure disorder (Hill, 1984). Approximately half the youngsters in the community sample were moderately to severely retarded.

Several surveys of community placements have now been conducted, and an accurate description of drug use is emerging. In Figure 3-5, the prevalence of antiepileptic drug use is presented from studies conducted in Illinois (Martin & Agran, 1985); Missouri (Intagliata & Rinck, 1985), Pennsylvania (Radinsky, 1984), the United States (Hill et al., 1983), and Auckland, New Zealand (Aman et al., 1985). The data from Illinois and New Zealand pertain only to adults (Martin & Agran, 1985; Aman et al., 1985).

Public Schools

In general, programs for trainable mentally retarded (TMR) pupils serve children and adolescents who score between 30/35 and 50/55 on standardized IQ tests. What is known about the pattern and prevalence of drug use among children in these programs comes from one statewide study conducted in Illinois (Gadow & Kalachnik, 1981), and one city-wide survey conducted in New Zealand (Aman et al., 1985).

The results of the Illinois study showed that 11.9% received medication for a seizure disorder at some time during the school year. This figure includes children who were receiving medication for both a behavior and a seizure disorder (1.8% of the sample were administered drugs for both disorders). Dilantin and phenobarbital were the two most frequently prescribed antiepileptic drugs, accounting for 62% of all seizure control medication (Table 3-3). The incidence rate for the onset of drug treatment for epilepsy during the school year was 3.9 new cases per 1,000. Parents reported the onset of treatment was usually quite early, often between birth and 2 years of age. Multiple-drug therapy was common, with well over half of the seizure-disordered children receiving more than one drug (see Fig. 3-2). Of that group of children, 26% took three or more drugs for seizure control.

Interestingly, the New Zealand prevalance data are similar. There, it was found that 17.4% of the "special school" children and adolescents were receiving antiepileptic medication.

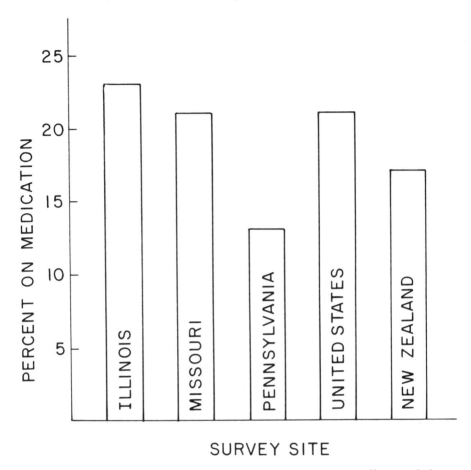

Figure 3-5. Prevalence of antiepileptic drug use for mentally retarded people in community placements as reported in five surveys.

Compared with the prevalence of antiepileptic drug treatment in residential facilities and community placements, pharmacotherapy for TMR children and adolescents in public school programs is much less frequent. However, both the relative frequency of the specific drugs prescribed for seizure management and the popularity of multiple-drug therapy are comparable across settings.

In general, children and adolescents who are referred to as educable mentally retarded (EMR) score between 50/55 and 75/80 on standardized IQ tests. Although recent efforts in mainstreaming have focused on EMR children, many remain in segregated programs for at least part of the school day (Borginsky, 1974; Epstein et

Table 3–3.   Drugs Prescribed for the Management of Seizure Disorders in Trainable Mentally Retarded Children

Generic Name	Trade Name	SD(N = 332)[a]	SD-BD(N = 60)[a]
Phenytoin	Dilantin	186	38
Phenobarbital		166	23
Primidone	Mysoline	62	10
Carbamazepine	Tegretol	26	3
Acetazolamide	Diamox	22	2
Ethosuximide	Zarontin	22	1
Clonazepam	Clonopin	19	1
Diazepam	Valium	18	3
Mephobarbital	Mebaral	13	1
Methsuximide	Celontin	7	4
Other		9	2
Unknown		19	3
Total[b]		569	91

Note: From "Prevalence and Pattern of Drug Treatment for Behavior and Seizure Disorders of TMR Students," by K. D. Gadow & J. Kalachnik, 1981, *American Journal of Mental Deficiency, 85,* p. 590. Copyright 1981 by the American Association on Mental Deficiency. Reprinted by permission.

[a] SD = on medication for seizure disorder; SD-BD = on medication for both behavior and seizure disorder.

[b] Totals are inflated because many children received two or more drugs during the school year.

al., 1985). Information about antiepileptic drug use for EMR students is not available, but it is generally believed that treatment prevalence rates are not that much different than those for nonretarded peers. Until more data are available, however, this remains a matter of speculation. Because the nature of the EMR population is changing (appears to be more seriously disabled) in the United States for a variety of reasons, the prevalence of antiepileptic drug therapy may be higher than in previous decades.

Issues Relating To Drug Treatment

Antiepileptic drug therapy with mentally retarded people has been the focus of some controversy for several reasons. First, research on the use of antiepileptic medication for mentally retarded people is very infrequent, and there have been few published accounts about how to improve the way in which pharmacotherapy is typically managed. Second, the manner in which these drugs are prescribed and administered (e.g., dosage, duration of treatment, monitoring) raises questions about possible drug misuse (e.g., Herberg, 1977;

Kaufman & Katz-Garris, 1979; O'Neill et al., 1977; Schain, 1975). Third, recent court cases involving residential facilities for mentally retarded persons have raised serious questions about the competence of caregivers. Some of the major issues in these court cases are overmedication, poor monitoring procedures, and a cavalier approach to recordkeeping on the use and effects of drugs. An excellent review of this material has been prepared by Sprague (1982). Fourth, the exclusion of teachers in public schools and of direct care personnel in residential facilities from meaningful participation in the treatment process is also a major problem (Gadow, 1982a, 1982b). Although antiepileptic drugs can affect the very behaviors that are targeted for educational and habilitative programming, nonmedical personnel are frequently excluded from drug evaluation procedures. Finally, because antiepileptics can produce serious side effects when used for long periods of time at high dosages and can suppress adaptive behavior, disagreements about the risk-to-benefit are unavoidable. Central to this issue is whether or not medication is being used in a manner that is in the best interest of the mentally retarded child.

These problems are, of course, highly interrelated and well known to many who have direct experience with residential facilities, and, to a lesser extent, public school special education programs. This is not to suggest that exemplary treatment evaluation programs do not exist because they do (e.g., O'Neill et al., 1977). This misuse of antiepileptic medication is often the product of inadequate training, incomplete medical knowledge, inappropriate diagnostic and drug assessment practices, and, in some cases, incompetence and societal irresponsibility.

The seriousness of poor monitoring procedures is evidenced in the following quote. Sprague (1977b), serving as an expert witness for the federal judiciary, was called upon to describe and evaluate procedures employed in residential facilities for mentally retarded children. He said in part:

> I made site visits to many of the private facilities for the Office of Special Litigation, and I found intolerable conditions for many of the children. In one facility for severely retarded children, the average stay for residents was 7.8 years with 66% of the residents receiving regular anticonvulsant medication. The monitoring of this medication was almost nonexistent in that the physician supervising these patients only ordered one laboratory test to check the physical effects of the medication once in 184.3 patient-years (a patient-year is one patient in the facility for one year). (p. 146)

The need for effective drug assessment procedures is self-evident to anyone who is concerned about the use of antiepileptic drugs with mentally retarded people. Almost all of the effort in this area is directed toward residential facilities because it is very difficult to either regulate or monitor drug use with children and adolescents in public schools for a variety of reasons. A number of articles have appeared in recent years that describe procedures to successfully reduce unnecessary antiepileptic drug use (e.g., O'Neill et al., 1977) and unnecessary multiple drug therapy (Bennett et al., 1983). One program is briefly described here to show how much can be done to improve the welfare of these often unfortunate people.

O'Neill et al. (1977) assessed the importance of monitoring blood levels of antiepileptic medication. Two years after instituting an interdisciplinary pilot program to improve health care for epileptic mentally retarded residents, researchers at the Lynchburg Training School and Hospital in Virginia reported notable changes. There was a significant reduction in toxic blood levels of anticonvulsant drugs, a 48% decrease in episodes of status epilepticus, and a 73% decrease in seizure-related deaths. As a result of improved monitoring procedures, 33% of the residents with uncontrolled seizures became seizure-free.

Another problem with antiepileptic drug treatment for mentally retarded people is the question of whether or not they are at greater risk for the development of certain side effects. Some examples are Dilantin-induced encephalopathy (a disease that produces a deterioration of brain function), characterized by decrease in psychomotor ability that improves somewhat with drug withdrawal (Meistrup-Larsen et al., 1979); cognitive deterioration as consequence of long-term treatment (e.g., Corbett et al., 1985); possible phenobarbital-induced behavior disorder (Gay, 1984); Dilantin-induced thickening of the skin of the mouth, nose, and forehead, which is referred to as *coarse facies* (Herberg, 1977; Lefebvre et al., 1972); and abnormally low levels of calcium in the blood (*hypocalcemia*) of institutionalized mentally retarded people receiving antiepileptic medication (see Livingston, 1978). Treatment with vitamin D appears to be of some help in treating drug-induced hypocalcemia (Hoikka et al., 1982). Dilantin-induced *gingival hyperplasia* can also be a greater problem for institutionalized people because "a soft diet, chronic neglect of oral hygiene and lethargy resulting from polypharmacy routinely elicit a high degree of gingival inflammation" (Hassell et al., 1984, p. 251).

While there have been reports that Depakene (valproic acid) is less useful with severely retarded children (Coulter et al., 1980), others have found it to be highly effective (Chayasirisobhon & Russell, 1983). Most of the reported cases of Depakene-induced liver toxicity have been in mentally retarded people (Jeavons, 1984), but fortunately this is a rare reaction. Depakene may have a beneficial cognitive effect for some institutionalized people with seizure disorders (Gay, 1984).

With mentally retarded people, it may be difficult to differentiate seizure phenomena and drug-induced behavioral toxicity from the person's regular behavior. Because institutionalized mentally retarded people exhibit a wide array of deviant behaviors and handicaps, diagnosis and drug monitoring is greatly complicated. Procedures such a videorecording behavior concurrent with EEG recording may help solve some diagnostic problems associated with certain types of seizure disorders (see Holmes et al., 1983).

Although much discussion has focused on private and public residential facilities, information collected about TMR children in public schools is equally discouraging. It was found that teachers received very little formal training regarding antiepileptic drugs even though they frequently encountered children on medication (Gadow, 1983). Nor were they provided basic information about the effects of medication on their students' behavior (Gadow, 1982a; Gadow & Kane, 1983). Interaction between school, parent, and physician was limited, and there was almost no direct contact between the teacher and doctor (Gadow, 1982b). Inadequate monitoring procedures were the result of poorly developed channels of communication, lack of standardized evaluation instruments, ambiguities in role behavior, and failure to establish routine drug evaluations. In general, teachers were excluded from what many epileptologists believe should be an interdisciplinary team effort. One cannot help but draw comparisons between the practices employed in some, but certainly not all, institutions and the situation that exists in the public schools.

SUGGESTED READINGS

Dreifuss, F. E. (1983). *Pediatric epileptology*. Littleton, MA: John Wright•PSG. (C, S)

Gadow, K. D. (1977). *Psychotropic and antiepileptic drug treatment with children in early childhood special education*. Champaign, IL: Institute for Child Behavior and Development, University of Illinois. (ERIC Document Reproduction Service No. ED 162 294) (C, S)

Gadow, K. D. (1982). School involvement in the treatment of seizure disorders. *Epilepsia, 23*, 215–224. (S)

Morselli, P. L., Pippenger, C. E., & Penry, J. K. (Eds.). (1983). *Antiepileptic drug therapy in pediatrics*. New York: Raven. (C, S)

REFERENCES

Aman, M. G., Field, C. J., & Bridgman, G. D. (1985). City-wide survey of drug patterns among noninstitutionalized retarded persons. *Applied Research in Mental Retardation, 6,* 159–171.

Bennett, H. S., Dunlop, T., & Ziring, P. (1983). Reduction of polypharmacy for epilepsy in an institution for the retarded. *Developmental Medicine and Child Neurology, 25,* 735–737.

Borginsky, M. E. (1974). *Provision of instruction to handicapped pupils in local public schools. Spring 1970.* Washington, DC: U.S. Office of Education.

Chayasirisobhon, S., & Russell, M. (1983). Valproic acid and intractable seizures in severely brain-damaged patients. *Neurology (NY), 33,* 99–101.

Cohen, M. N., & Sprague, R. L. (1977, March). *Survey of drug usage in two midwestern institutions for the retarded.* Paper presented at the Gatlinburg Conference on Research in Mental Retardation, Gatlinburg, TN.

Corbett, J. A., Trimble, M. R., & Nichol, T. C. (1985). Behavioral and cognitive impairments in children with epilepsy: The long-term effects of anticonvulsant therapy. *Journal of the American Academy of Child Psychiatry, 24,* 17–23.

Cordes, C. K. (1973). Chronic drug intoxication causing pseudo-retardation in a young child. *Journal of the American Academy of Child Psychiatry, 12,* 215–222.

Coulter, D. L., Wu, H., & Allen, R. J. (1980). Valproic acid therapy in childhood epilepsy. *Journal of the American Medical Association, 244,* 785–788.

Dekaban, A. S., & Lehman, E. J. B. (1975). Effects of different dosages of anticonvulsant drugs on mental performance in patients with chronic epilepsy. *Acta Neurologica Scandinavica, 52,* 319–330.

Dreifuss, F. E. (1983). *Pediatric epileptology.* Littleton, MA: John Wright•PSG.

Epstein, M. H., Cullinan, D., & Gadow, K. D. (1985). *Prevalence of psychotropic drug use with learning disabled, emotionally disturbed, and mentally retarded children.* Unpublished manuscript, Northern Illinois University, Department of Learning Development, and Special Education, DeKalb.

Gadow, K. D. (1975, October). *Pills and preschool: Medication usage with young children in special education.* Paper presented at the Illinois Council for Exceptional Children, Chicago, October.

Gadow, K. D. (1977). *Psychotropic and antiepileptic drug treatment with children in early childhood special education.* Champaign, IL: Institute for Child Behavior and Development, University of Illinois. (ERIC Document Reproduction Service No. ED 162 294)

Gadow, K. D. (1982a). Problems with students on medication. *Exceptional Children, 49,* 20–27.

Gadow, K. D. (1982b). School involvement in the treatment of seizure disorders. *Epilepsia, 23,* 215–224.

Gadow, K. D. (1983). Educating teachers about pharmacotherapy. *Education and Training of the Mentally Retarded, 18,* 69–73.

Gadow, K. D., & Kalachnik, J. (1981). Prevalence and pattern of drug treatment for behavior and seizure disorders of TMR students. *American Journal of Mental Deficiency, 85,* 588–595.

Gadow, K. D., & Kane, K. M. (1983). Administration of medication by school personnel. *Journal of School Health, 53,* 178–183.

Gay, P. E. (1984). Effects of antiepileptic drugs and seizure type on operant responding in mentally retarded persons. *Epilepsia, 25,* 377–386.

Hassell, T., O'Donnell, J., Pearlman, J., Tesini, D., Murphy, T., & Best, H. (1984). Phenytoin induced gingival overgrowth in institutionalized epileptics. *Journal of Clinical Periodontology, 11,* 242–253.

Herberg, K. P. (1977). Effects of diphenylhydantoin in 41 epileptics institutionalized since childhood. *Southern Medical Journal, 70,* 19–24.

Hill, B. (1984). Personal communication, November 26.

Hill, B. K., Balow, E. A., & Bruininks, R. H. (1983). *A national study of prescribed drugs in institutions and community residential facilities for mentally retarded people* (Brief No. 20). Minneapolis: University of Minnesota, Department of Educational Psychology.

Hill, B. K., Lakin, K. C., & Bruininks, R. H. (1984). Trends in residential services for people who are mentally retarded: 1977–1982. *Journal of the Association for Persons with Severe Handicaps, 9,* 243–250.

Hoikka, V., Savolainen, K., Karjalainen, P., Alhava, E. M., & Sivenius, S. (1982). Treatment of osteomalacia in institutionalized epileptic patients on long-term anticonvulsant therapy. *Annals of Clinical Research, 14,* 72–75.

Holmes, G. L., McKeever, M., & Russman, B. S. (1983). Abnormal behavior or epilepsy? Use of long-term EEG and video monitoring with severely to profoundly mentally retarded patients with seizures. *American Journal of Mental Deficiency, 87,* 456–458.

Intagliata, J., & Rinck, C. (1985). Psychoactive drug use in public and community residential facilities for mentally retarded persons. *Psychopharmacology Bulletin, 21,* 268–278.

Jasper, H. H., Ward, A. A., & Pope, A. (Eds.). *Basic mechanisms of the epilepsies.* Boston: Little, Brown.

Jeavons, P. M. (1984). Non-dose-related side effects of valproate. *Epilepsia* (Suppl. 1), S50–S55.

Kaufman, K. R., & Katz-Garris, L. (1979). Epilepsy, mental retardation, and anticonvulsant therapy. *American Journal of Mental Deficiency, 84,* 256–259.

Kirman, B. (1975). Drug therapy in mental handicap. *British Journal of Psychiatry, 127,* 545–549.

Lefebvre, E. B., Haining, R. G., & Labbe, F. F. (1972). Coarse facies, calverial thickening and hyperphosphatasia associated with long-term anticonvulsant therapy. *New England Journal of Medicine, 286,* 1301–1302.

Livingston, S. (1972). *Comprehensive management of epilepsy in infancy, childhood and adolescence.* Springfield, IL: Charles C Thomas.

Livingston, S. (1978). Medical treatment of epilepsy: Part II. *Southern Medical Journal, 71,* 432–447.

Martin, J. E., & Agran, M. (1985). Psychotropic and anticonvulsant drug use by mentally retarded adults across community residential and vocational placements. *Applied Research in Mental Retardation, 6,* 33–49.

Meistrup-Larsen, K. I., Hermann, S., & Permin, H. (1979). Chronic diphen-ylhydantoin encephalopathy in mentally retarded children and adoles-cent with severe epilepsy. *Acta Neurologica Scandinavica, 60,* 50–55.

Morselli, P. L., Pippenger, C. E., & Penry, J. K. (Eds.). (1983). *Antiepileptic drug therapy in pediatrics.* New York: Raven.

O'Neill, B. P., Ladon, B., Harris, L. M., Riley, H. L., & Dreifuss, F. E. (1977). A comprehensive, interdisciplinary approach to the care of the institu-tionalized person with epilepsy. *Epilepsia, 18,* 243–250.

Payne, D., Johnson, R. C., & Abelson, R. B. (1969). *Comprehensive descrip-tion of institutionalized retardates in Western United States.* Boulder, CO: Western Interstate Commission for Higher Education.

Pulman, R. M., Pook, R. B., & Singh, N. N. (1979). Prevalence of drug therapy for institutionalized mentally retarded children. *Australian Journal of Mental Retardation, 5,* 212–214.

Radinsky, A. M. (1984). *A descriptive study of psychotropic and antiepilep-tic medication use with mentally retarded persons in three residential environments.* Unpublished doctoral dissertation, University of Pitts-burgh.

Schain, R. J. (1975, May). *Problems in the use of anticonvulsant drugs in the mentally retarded.* Paper presented at the Workshop on Psychotro-pic Drugs and the Mentally Retarded at the meeting of the American Association on Mental Deficiency, Portland, Oregon.

Silva, D. A. (1979). The use of medication in a residential institution for mentally retarded persons. *Mental Retardation, 17,* 285–288.

Slater, E., & Cowie, V. (1971). *The genetics of mental disorders.* London: Oxford University Press.

Spencer, D. A. (1974). A survey of the medication in a hospital for the mentally handicapped. *British Journal of Psychiatry, 124,* 507–508.

Sprague, R. L. (1977a). Overview of psychopharmacology for the retarded in the United States. In P. Mittler (Ed.), *Research to practice in mental retardation* (Vol. 3, pp. 199–202). Baltimore: University Park Press.

Sprague, R. L. (1977b). Psychopharmacotherapy in children. In M. F. McMillan & S. Henao (Eds.), *Child psychiatry: Treatment and research* (pp. 130–149). New York: Brunner/Mazel.

Sprague, R. L. (1982). Litigation, legislation, and regulations. In S. E. Breuning & A. D. Poling (Eds.), *Drugs and mental retardation* (pp. 377–414). Springfield, IL: Charles C Thomas.

Svensmark, O., & Buchthal, F. (1964). Diphenylhydantoin and phenobarbi-tal: Serum levels in children. *American Journal of Diseases of Chil-dren, 108,* 82–87.

Tu, J. B. (1979). A survey of psychotropic medication in mental retardation facilities. *Journal of Clinical Psychiatry, 40,* 125–128.

Wilson, J. (1969). Drug treatment of epilepsy in childhood. *British Medical Journal, 4,* 475–477.

Chapter 4

Emotional Disturbance

Perhaps one of the most ambiguous labels to ever emerge from the childhood psychopathology literature is *emotional disturbance*. In child psychiatry, particularly during the 1950s and 1960s, the term was used in drug studies to refer to heterogeneous groups of children and adolescents who were housed in psychiatric hospitals or residential facilities (e.g., Bender & Nichtern, 1956; Conners et al., 1964) or who were outpatients in a psychiatric or child guidance clinic (e.g., Freed & Peifer, 1956). Although investigators often diagnosed each child in a sample as exhibiting a specific psychiatric disorder (e.g., primary behavior disorder, psychoneurotic, schizophrenic, reactive behavior disorder with organic brain disease; see Freed & Peifer, 1956), not everyone agreed as to what disorders should be considered emotional disturbance. Moreover, in many of the early studies drug response (which was often evaluated and described in a vague and imprecise manner) was rarely analyzed with regard to specific disorders or behavioral symptoms. There were, of course, notable exceptions (e.g., Conners et al., 1964). In addition, the diagnostic constructs themselves were poorly operationalized and have undergone revisions over the years, rendering many of these earlier studies uninterpretable with regard to current perspectives. Interestingly, according to the *Diagnostic and Statistical Manual of Mental Disorders* published by the American Psychiatric Association (1980), only the anxiety disorders and a few other conditions (e.g., schizoid disorder, elective mutism, oppositional disorder) are classified as "emotional" disorders (p. 36).

If the study sample was selected from children enrolled in special education classes for children labeled emotionally disturbed, the situation is even more bizarre because the educational research community has made little or no effort to identify diagnostic categories to either (a) assess response to educational interventions, (b) evaluate the residual benefits of treatment, (c) describe the natural history of a condition, (d) identify potential etiological mechanisms, or (e) to examine prevalence and distribution. Therefore, it is unclear exactly what conclusions can be drawn from samples of emotionally disturbed school children, unless the investigator selected a particular type of child. For all the aforementioned reasons, it is meaningless to talk about drug therapy for emotional disturbance.

Before describing psychotropic drug use for various psychiatric disorders that are found with relative frequency in children who are labeled emotionally disturbed by our schools, it may be useful to explain the educator's perspective. To begin with, for a child to be labeled emotionally disturbed in the United States, he or she must meet the requirements implied in the definition specified in Public Law 94–142, which are as follows:

> The term [seriously emotionally disturbed] means a condition exhibiting one or more of the following characteristics over a long period of time and to a marked degree, which adversely affects educational performance: (a) an inability to learn which cannot be explained by intellectual, sensory, or health factors; (b) an inability to build or maintain satisfactory interpersonal relationships with peers and teachers; (c) inappropriate types of behavior or feelings under normal circumstances; (d) a general pervasive mood of unhappiness or depression; or (e) a tendency to develop physical symptoms or fears associated with personal or school problems. The term includes children who are schizophrenic or autistic. The term does not include children who are socially maladjusted, unless it is determined that they are seriously emotionally disturbed. (Federal Register, 1977, 42, p. 42478)

There are a number of problems associated with this special education categorical construct, just three of which are noted here. One, the use of the qualifier "seriously" suggests that the educational rights of children with mild to moderate behavior disorders are not protected by federal law (see Raiser & Van Nagel, 1980). This is obviously unfortunate because there are no doubt many hyperactive and hyperactive-aggressive children, for example, who could benefit from behavior modification programs within the regular classroom if the teacher had access to trained professionals, which could be made mandatory as a result of federal law.

Second, the diagnostic criteria for what constitutes emotional disturbance are sufficiently vague as to create conflict among caregivers as to whom should be considered emotionally disturbed (see, for example, Kammerlohr et al., 1983). Some have inferred, for example, that the exclusion of socially maladjusted children (who are not also seriously emotionally disturbed) implies that youngsters with conduct problems are excluded from consideration for special education.

A third problem pertains to the label itself, which is offensive and misleading to many people, particularly parents. This is attested to by the fact that many states have adopted the term *behavior disordered* (or some variant) as a substitute for the label emotionally disturbed (see Bricklin & Gallico, 1984). Furthermore, it is unclear exactly whose emotions are disturbed, the child's or his or her caregivers' (see Algozzine, 1977). In other words, although the behavior of school-labeled emotionally disturbed youngsters may disturb our emotional state by making us frustrated and angry, it does not follow that their emotions are necessarily disturbed. We see many parents in our Child Psychiatry Clinic who are referred to us by their local school district and who are confused by this terminology. Many recognize full well that their child is aggressive, hyperactive, and difficult to manage, but cannot understand what any of that has to do with emotional disturbance. This is related to another conceptual difficulty, namely, intrapsychic conflict. The term *emotional disturbance* as it is used by the educational establishment implies to some caregivers that the manifest behavior is the result of a mental conflict that possibly stems from an unresolved psychological trauma that can only be corrected by an in-depth analysis of the child's feelings. Although stressful events (e.g., death in the family, parental divorce) can and do lead to aberrant behavior, this is not necessarily the case, as is evidenced by the literally millions of school children who do experience such stressors and are never labeled emotionally disturbed (but who *may* nevertheless have temporary episodes of distress). The notion that intrapsychic conflict is a common cause of aberrant behavior appears to be a widely held and deeply entrenched belief in the education establishment. The fact that many school-identified emotionally disturbed children elicit inappropriately intense emotional reactions (e.g., tantrums, explosive outbursts, whining, and so forth) probably reinforces this belief to some extent.

Although it is pointless to discuss the prevalence of emotional disturbance for reasons already noted, it is a simple matter to determine the number of children labeled emotionally disturbed (or equivalent label). Because two laws (Public Law 89–313 and Public Law 94–142) require states to report to the federal government the number of children between the ages of 3 and 21 years who are receiving special education services, it is possible to obtain fairly accurate figures for school-labeled emotionally disturbed (or equivalent label) students in the United States. Public 94–142 pertains to children receiving special education and other services primarily in public school classes, whereas Public Law 89–313 refers to children in state-operated and/or state-supported schools that receive federal funds. There were 320,599 and 41,474 children reported under these two laws, respectively, in December, 1983. Emotional disturbance accounts for 6 to 8% of all handicapped students, a figure that has remained fairly constant for at least several years. On a national level, approximately 1% of all school children are labeled emotionally disturbed.

Because few people have ever attempted to examine large samples of school-identified emotionally disturbed children with regard to psychiatric diagnoses, it is extremely difficult to integrate the educational and medical literature on these children. Nevertheless, on the basis of published findings from behavior rating scale studies (e.g., Cullinan et al., 1984, McCarthy & Paraskevopoulos, 1969; Quay et al., 1966) and clinical experience, it is possible to generate a list of childhood psychiatric disorders that are fairly common in this population of school children and that may be treated with medication. It is important to emphasize that all the disorders described here range in seriousness from mild to severe and that medication rarely cures the disorder. In addition, behavioral symptoms are not static. They often improve over the course of time, even during a single school year. Therefore, although drug treatment prevalence rates for school-labeled emotionally disturbed children are relatively high (15 to 30%; see Epstein et al., 1985; Safer & Krager, 1984), most do not take psychotropic medication.

The drug-treated disorders that are most likely to land a child in a special education program for emotionally disturbed youngsters are severe hyperactivity (often with pronounced aggression or noncompliance), aggressivity (conduct disorder, undersocialized aggressive), psychosis (infantile autism, childhood schizophrenia), and possibly affective disorders (e.g., childhood depression). This chapter focuses on some of the more severe forms of aberrant behavior, with each disorder presented in alphabetical order. Unfortunately, it was possible to give only passing mention to diagnostic issues and nondrug therapies. Because the majority of drug-treated hyperactive children are not placed in classes for the emotionally disturbed (Safer & Krager, 1984), this condition is not discussed here (see the companion volume).

The neuroleptics are among the most commonly prescribed agents for severe behavior disorders and childhood psychoses and have been used to treat almost all childhood and adolescent psychiatric disorders. Therefore, to avoid repetition, it seemed instructive to present an overview of this class of drugs as an introduction to the treatment of these disabilities. Because the question of clinical efficacy is addressed for each condition, the overview focuses more on general drug effects. It must be emphasized that the role of these and other psychotropic agents in the treatment process has always been recognized as being an adjunctive one. In one of the earliest reviews of the use of neuroleptics and antianxiety agents with children, Charles Bradley (1958) noted that:

> A major objective for the use of pharmacotherapy of children with behavior problems is to enable them to be free of disturbing symptoms for a period long enough to permit them to build up confidence in themselves. To insure this objective, the use of medication must always be accompanied by other available forms of guidance and psychologic management. (p. 334)

NEUROLEPTICS: GENERAL TOPICS

The first report of the use of a neuroleptic (Thorazine) in the treatment of adult psychiatric disorders appeared in 1952. A year later, the first article about the use of Thorazine (known as Largactil in Europe and Canada) with children was published (Heuyer et al., 1953). Since then, literally dozens of neuroleptics have been developed and marketed. A listing of many of these agents appears in Appendix A. Although it would seem that ample time has elapsed to collect a considerable amount of research information about the effects of these agents in children, relatively few studies have actually been conducted (see Aman, 1984; Aman & Singh, 1983; DiMascio et al., 1970; Sprague & Werry, 1974). Much of what has been done contains serious methodological flaws and lacks systematic documentation of side effects.

This section describes neuroleptic drug effects in adults. Although this may sound at odds with the primary focus of this text, there are really three good reasons for so doing. One, the distinction between late adolescence and adulthood is probably not an important one in terms of drug response. Two, many treatment-related issues are similar for all age groups. Three, in contrast to pediatric research, there is a voluminous literature about the use of neuroleptics in the treatment of adult psychiatric disorders.

The neuroleptics consist primarily of three subgroups of drugs: *phenothiazines* (e.g., Mellaril, Thorazine, Stelazine), *butyrophenones* (e.g., Haldol), and *thioxanthenes* (e.g., Taractan, Navane). The phenothiazines are the most widely used neuroleptics and, for this reason, they are the primary focus of the following discussion. There are two more categories of neuroleptics (see Appendix A) but at present, they are used infrequently with children and adolescents. Although there are some marked differences in the prevalence of certain adverse drug reactions, all the neuroleptics have similar effects on behavior disorders. They have proved to be effective in the suppression of some symptoms associated with certain psychiatric disorders such as schizophrenia, character disorders, manic states, and agitated depression (Klein et al., 1980). These drugs can have a pronounced effect on disordered thought, hyperactive behavior, combativeness, and uncooperativeness. Patients who suffer dramatic changes in mood in a relatively short period of time are also aided by these agents because of their mood-regulating effects. Other therapeutic benefits for schizophrenic patients include making them less withdrawn and more responsive and suppressing hallucinations and delusions.

The general behavioral effects of the phenothiazines in psychiatric patients are "suppression of spontaneous movements and complex behavior . . . a striking lack of initiative, disinterest in the environment, little display of emotion, and limited range of affect" (Baldessarini, 1980, p. 397). To an observer, adults receiving phenothiazines are not upset by situations or events that would normally arouse them, perceiving the world with a detached serenity. Although fully capable of thinking clearly and conversing, they appear indifferent to feelings and express thoughts without emotion. Spontaneous motor activity can be greatly reduced. People taking phenothiazines perform less well on tasks that require sustained attention, and there is a general impairment in cognitive performance and learning at higher dosages (Hartlage, 1965). Initially, Mellaril (thioridazine) and Thorazine (chlorpromazine) produce a considerable degree of sedation (drowsiness, lethargy) for which the patient usually develops a tolerance within several days to a few weeks, often without a reduction in dosage.

Side Effects

In addition to their ability to alter mood, thought processes, and behavior, phenothiazines affect a number of bodily functions (Baldessarini, 1980; Klein et al., 1980). They produce a variety of autonomic nervous system reactions that include blurred vision, dry mouth, nausea, decreased sweating and salivation, nasal stuffiness, dizziness, constipation, and inhibition of ejaculation (but may not interfere with erection). The latter is particularly true of Mellaril. Another common autonomic nervous system side effect is *orthostatic hypotension*, which refers to lowered blood pressure upon standing erect. Persons experiencing such a reaction may feel faint, dizzy, or weak, especially when they get up in the morning. It usually appears during the first week of treatment but is seldom a problem because tolerance for this reaction develops rather quickly.

The endocrine system can also be affected by treatment with the phenothiazines. Drug-induced changes in the release of growth hormones may account for frequent reports of increased appetite and weight gain.

Jaundice is observed in less than 2 to 4% of the patients treated with Thorazine. Other estimates, however, put the prevalence of this reaction at less than 1% (Klein et al., 1980). This is generally mild and commonly occurs between the second and fourth week of treatment. If jaundice occurs, treatment is usually terminated and another drug is substituted.

Skin reactions are fairly common, with *urticaria* or *dermatitis* reported in about 5% of those treated with phenothiazines. This usually occurs within the first to fifth week of treatment, clearing up when medication is discontinued. Most skin rashes are *self-limiting* (disappear with time).

Phototoxicity is another type of skin reaction. In some people taking phenothiazines, exposure to the sun for even a few minutes results in a severe sunburn. This can be prevented by simply keeping clothed areas well covered and using a sunscreen on skin exposed to sunlight. Long-term drug use at high dosages can also produce a gray-blue pigmentation in skin areas exposed to the sun.

Neuroleptics, particularly high doses or rapid increases in dosage, can cause tonic-clonic (grand mal) seizures. This can be easily managed by making a slight decrease in dosage.

After reviewing the psychiatric literature, Klein and Davis (1969) classified the frequency of side effects as very frequent (20% or more), frequent (10 to 20%), and occasional (5 to 10%). For Mellaril, the very frequent side effects were nausea, vomiting, drowsiness, dizziness, and dry mouth. Frequent adverse effects were visual disturbance and constipation; occasionally, patients were confused or had urinary disturbance. The very frequent side effects of Thorazine were drowsiness, dry mouth, and weight increase. Frequent effects were depression, visual disturbance, and constipation; occasional effects include confusion, allergic reactions, and endocrine disturbances.

Extrapyramidal Syndromes

Perhaps the most disquieting and alarming side effects of neuroleptics are the *extrapyramidal syndromes*. These are disorders that involve certain motor areas of the brain called the *extrapyramidal tract*. The various *nuclei* (groups of nerve cells) and nerve fibers that make up this structure control and coordinate motor activities, especially walking, posture, muscle tone, and patterns of movement. Drugs that affect the extrapyramidal tract can cause spasms in skeletal muscles and changes in body posture, facial expression, and movement of the limbs. Four different extrapyramidal syndromes are associated with the use of major tranquilizers: *Parkinsonian syndrome, akathisia, acute dystonic reactions,* and *tardive dyskinesia.* These side effects are most common in treatment with Haldol (haloperidol), Stelazine (trifluoperazine), and Compazine (prochlorperazine) and are less least likely to occur with Mellaril (see Table 5–3 in the chapter on adolescent disorders).

Parkinsonian Syndrome. The Parkinsonian syndrome caused by the neuroleptics appears similar to the symptoms of Parkinson's disease. The syndrome is characterized by a decrease in spontaneous movements. The patient may appear depressed, with a masklike facial expression that parents and other caregivers may refer to as "looking like a zombie." Associated with this is muscle rigidity, changes in posture, and *tremor* (involuntary shaking, trembling, or quivering). Other features may include drooling, a shuffling walk without free swing of the arms, and "pill-rolling." The latter refers to movements of the hand as if the patient is rolling a pill between his or her fingers. There is disagreement as to the best way of managing this side effect. Some patients may respond to dosage reduction, whereas others may require *anticholinergic* agents, such as Artane (trihexyphenidyl) or Cogentin (benztropine). For children, oral doses of 1 mg of Artane three times a day or 1 to 2 mg of Cogentin three times a day rapidly alleviate these symptoms (Winsberg et al., 1976).

Akathisia. This reaction is characterized by involuntary motor restlessness. The patient is unable to sit still, is constantly fidgeting, and appears to be agitated. The disorder responds to dosage reduction and in some cases anticholinergic drugs.

Acute Dystonic Reaction. A third type of extrapyramidal syndrome is acute dystonic reaction. Symptoms include one or more of the following: facial grimacing, *oculogyric crisis* (fixed upward gaze), and *torticollis* (a twisting of the neck and an unnatural positioning of the head due to contraction of the neck muscles). The tongue may be protruded or the teeth tightly clenched. In rare cases, the patient may have difficulty swallowing. Although this reaction responds well to treatment, it can be terrifying for both patient and caregivers. Acute dystonic reactions are common with Compazine and Stelazine compared with the other neuroleptics. They are more apt to occur in younger patients and when medication is first initiated. A child having a severe reaction should receive immediate medical attention. The physician may use an intramuscular injection of Benadryl (diphenhydramine) or of anticholinergic agents for immediate relief of symptoms, and later prescribe oral doses of Cogentin or Artane for the continued control of this reaction.

Tardive Dyskinesia. The fourth extrapyramidal syndrome, tardive dyskinesia, typically appears late, often months after drug treatment has been initiated, and may not be evident until medication is discontinued. Tardive dyskinesia is characterized by rhythmic, repetitive stereotyped movements that appear to be involuntary but can usually be inhibited. Some of the major features are sucking and smacking movements of the lips and side-to-side shifts of the chin, giving the appearance of a cow "chewing its cud." The tongue may dart in and out in a "fly-catching" fashion. Other symptoms include a sudden flying of the arms, up-and-down movement of the toes, in and out movements of the fingers or "piano playing," and jerky body movements. (See Kalachnik, 1985, for a detailed description of the syndrome.) Tardive dyskinesia is more common among patients who receive large dosages of neuroleptic medication over extended periods. Prevalence figures for this adverse reaction range as high as 15 to 30% among psychiatric patients. There is no one best method for treating tardive dyskinesia (Kobayashi, 1977). When the disorder appears while the person is on medication, treatment should be stopped, if possible, or another agent selected if drug therapy is necessary. For individuals who develop the disorder after treatment has been terminated, a variety of drugs that have helped some people are available. Other patients are benefited by resuming the drug that caused the tardive dyskinesia. The disorder can persist indefinitely after medication is terminated, but for at least half the patients, there is gradual improvement over time after medication has been stopped. Some very preliminary data suggest that gradual neuroleptic drug withdrawal in mentally retarded people produces fewer dyskinesias than abrupt drug withdrawal (Schroeder & Gualtieri, 1985).

Several large studies of drug treatment with psychotic, emotionally disturbed, and mentally retarded children have clearly documented tardive dyskinesia in children (McAndrew et al., 1972; Paulson et al., 1975; Polizos et al., 1973). Involuntary movements of the lips, tongue, and jaw are much less common among children than adults. Choreiform (ceaseless, rapid, and jerky involuntary) movements of the arms, legs, and head were the most frequently reported symptoms in children with tardive dyskinesia. For many children, the syndrome did not become apparent until medication was terminated. Off medication, some children improved over time and others became worse. Resuming drug treatment alleviated symptoms in many children who remained unchanged or became worse when treatment was stopped. McAndrew et al. (1972) reported that tardive dyskinesia was more common among children who received higher dosages for longer periods of time than among children on short-term regimens at lower dosages.

Children Versus Adults. There are some general differences between children and adults in the prevalence of extrapyramidal reactions (Winsberg & Yepes, 1978). The Parkinsonian syndrome is most common among older adult patients and is not often observed in children. When it does occur in children, the reaction is usually mild. Acute dystonic reactions are found more often in children and appear within 24 to 72 hours after the onset of treatment. The most common extrapyramidal syndrome in adults is akathisia, which is typically seen in middle-aged women. It is also reported in children, but the prevalence rate is difficult to determine. Tardive dyskinesia seems to occur with similar frequency in both children and adults, especially at higher doses. In one study of schizophrenic children receiving neuroleptics at doses comparable with those recommended for adults, 48% exhibited neurological symptoms similar to those of tardive dyskinesia upon withdrawal of medication (Engelhardt et al., 1975).

NEUROLEPTICS: PREPUBERTAL CHILDREN

There has been very little research on the use of neuroleptics with children and adolescents since the late 1950s and early 1960s when these drugs were first becoming widely used. These early studies were often, but not always, poorly done, at least according to contemporary standards. Subsequently, much of what has been written about the use of these agents with prepubertal children has been extrapolated from research and clinical experience with adolescents and adults. In addition, many of the truly well-designed studies have been conducted with hyperactive children (e.g., Gittelman-Klein et al., 1976; Sprague et al., 1970; Werry & Aman, 1975).

Side Effects

Side effects of neuroleptics in children are similar to those reported for adults. Sedative effects (drowsiness, lethargy, apathy) are quite common with Thorazine, but children usually develop a tolerance for this reaction within several days to a few weeks. Dosage reduction may be necessary in some cases. It is noteworthy that irritability and excitability are also possible. Skin reactions are infrequent. Also reported are diarrhea, upset stomach, dry mouth, blurred vision, constipation, urinary retention, and abdominal pain (Winsberg & Yepes, 1978). A number of studies reported increased appetite, weight gain, or both, during drug treatment.

Side effects are believed to be less frequent with Mellaril than with Thorazine. Adverse drug reactions commonly associated with Mellaril are drowsiness, lethargy, irritability, hyperactivity, ataxia, and dizziness. Increased appetite and weight gain are also not unusual. Because Mellaril has been reported to have a favorable effect on seizure reduction, this drug can be used with some confidence for the treatment of behavior disorders in epileptic children (Kamm & Mandel, 1967).

Katz et al. (1975) stated that in their experience with hyperactive children the side effects of Mellaril were frequent and severe. Drowsiness was the most common adverse reaction that was difficult to manage. If the dose was reduced, the drowsiness was less severe, but the therapeutic response was weaker. Many children developed enuresis and had to be taken off medication. Increased appetite was also common, as was puffiness around the eyes and mild dry mouth. Stomachache, nausea, and vomiting necessitated dosage reduction in a number of children. Other side effects included nosebleed, mild tremor, and orthostatic hypotension. Some children who reacted well to Mellaril later developed changes in temperament: They became irritable, moody, and belligerent, and medication eventually had to be stopped.

Extrapyramidal syndromes are frequently reported in studies using Haldol to control behavior disorders in children. Clinicians manage these side effects by either administering an anticholinergic agent at the beginning of drug treatment (a practice that is controversial), after symptoms appear, or after the discontinuation of treatment. Although Haldol is usually not associated with sedative effects (see Table 4–1), drowsiness was sometimes reported in studies with children. Other side effects include nausea, ataxia, slurred speech, and weight gain.

Perhaps the most controversial side effect of neuroleptics is cognitive and academic impairment. This is controversial because the studies in this area are not particularly laudatory (see Aman, 1984). There are, nevertheless, good examples of research with neuroleptics in nonretarded (e.g., Sprague et al., 1970; Werry & Aman, 1975) and mentally retarded (e.g., Wysocki et al., 1981) individuals that strongly suggest that mental impairment is a definite *possibility*. It is important, therefore, to monitor adaptive behavior during dosage adjustment to assess the extent to which desirable behaviors may be adversely affected

Dosage

There is a considerable range in reported dosages across drug studies with children and some general guidelines for children between 6 and 12 years old are presented in Table 4–1. It is important to note, however, that some of these neuroleptics are not approved for use with prepubertal children in the United States. The dose for Thorazine and Mellaril ranges from 10 to 1,000 mg per day, with an average daily dose of 75 to 200 mg. Some clinicians prescribe one large dose at night to avoid daytime drowsiness, whereas others divide the total amount into two or three doses during the day (Katz et al., 1975; Winsberg et al., 1976). Most hyperactive children require no more than 50 to 100 mg three times per day. Relative to body weight, the average dose is 3 to 6 mg/kg per day. The effective dose of Haldol ranges from 2 to 5 mg per day, which is divided into three daily doses. It is noteworthy that significant improvements in cognitive performance have been reported with doses of Haldol as low as

Table 4-1. Neuroleptic Drug Dosages for Children under 12 Years of Age[a]

Trade Name	Generic Name	Oral Dose (mg/day)
Haldol	haloperidol	0.25–16
Mellaril	thioridazine	10–200
Moban[b]	molindone	1–40
Navane[b]	thiothixene	1–40
Orap[c]	pimozide	1–7
Prolixin[b]	fluphenazine	0.25–16
Stelazine[d]	trifluoperazine	1–20
Thorazine	chlorpromazine	10–200

[a]The most current issue of the *Physicians' Desk Reference* should be consulted for dosage information.

[b]As of 1985, not approved by the Food and Drug Administration in the United States for use with children under 12 years of age.

[c]Approved for use in the pediatric age range only for the treatment of Tourette syndrome.

[d]Recommended for use only with children who are hospitalized or under close supervision.

0.025 mg/kg in nonretarded hyperactive boys (Werry & Aman, 1975). Daily doses for Stelazine range from 2 mg to 50 mg per day, with an average of 6 to 15 mg per day. In most studies, medication is given in divided doses, usually three times per day.

Monitoring for Tardive Dyskinesia

Tardive dyskinesia, or TD, has become an important issue in hospitals and residential facilities for several reasons: (a) high neuroleptic drug exposure in terms of prevalence, dosage, and duration of treatment (see Gualtieri et al., 1984), (b) inadequate side effect monitoring systems, and (c) a flurry of recent court cases (see Kalachnik, 1985). For patients in residential facilities who must receive neuroleptic medication, the most prudent course of action for caregivers is the development of a TD monitoring system. Several are described in the professional literature (e.g., Kalachnik, 1985; Kalachnik et al., 1983, 1984; Glazer & Moore, 1981; Whall et al., 1983). There are also several TD assessment scales, two of the more popular are the Abnormal Involuntary Movement Scale (Guy, 1976) and the Dyskinesia Identification System-Coldwater (Sprague et al., 1984a, 1984b). The latter (which is called DIS-Co) appears in Appendix E and item descriptions are given in Appendix F. An abbreviated version (DISCUS) is presented in Appendix G, the manual for which can be obtained from Sprague et al. (1985).

AUTISM (INFANTILE)

Infantile autism is a rare disorder affecting 2 to 4 children in every 10,000 (e.g., Gillberg, 1984). It is, nevertheless, a widely known and frequently discussed conditi n. The key features are a lack of responsiveness to other people, which is called *autism*, serious speech abnormalities (e.g., *echolalia*, improper use of pronouns, lack of speech, inability to use abstractions), and bizarre mannerisms (resistance to change in the environment, emotional attachment to strange objects, *stereotypies*), all of which must be exhibited before 30 months of age (hence, it is sometimes referred to as *early infantile autism*). The characteristic diagnostic features are presented in Table 4–2. Most, but certainly not all, children who have infantile autism score in the mentally retarded range on standardized intelligence tests (Gillberg, 1984), although some youngsters possess extraordinary mental abilities. The disorder is much more common in boys and is chronic in nature; in other words, it is a lifelong disability. Although some autistic children are able to achieve economic self-sufficiency in adulthood, the majority either suffer from the residual effects of the condition (social ineptness) or are provided for in institutional facilities or community placements (e.g., sheltered workshop). When an individual who was diagnosed as autistic improves and no longer meets all the original diagnostic criteria but still experiences some problems, the condition is known as *Infantile autism, residual state* (American Psychiatric Association, 1980). Those with higher intellectual ability and better language skills enjoy a more favorable prognosis. Seizure disorders may emerge during adolescence or adulthood.

Drug Therapy

Because infantile autism is so difficult to treat, it is not an exaggeration to say that almost every psychotropic and antiepileptic drug has been administered to this population. At present, no drugs "cure" this disorder, but symptom suppression is achieved in some cases. Fish (1976) described the role of medication in treatment as follows:

> I believe that any child with a disorder as serious as autism deserves a trial of drug treatment. Only in much milder psychiatric conditions can social and educational measures completely resolve the symptoms and return the patient to normal functioning. (p. 108)

There are several excellent reviews on this topic (Campbell & Deutsch, 1985; Campbell et al., 1981, 1984a; Fish, 1976). The following material is summarized from these articles.

Table 4–2. DSM III Diagnostic Criteria for Infantile Autism[a]

1. Onset before 30 months of age.
2. Pervasive lack of responsiveness to other people (autism).
3. Gross deficits in language development.
4. If speech is present, peculiar speech patterns such as immediate and delayed echolalia, metaphorical language, pronominal reversal.
5. Bizarre responses to various aspects of the environment, e.g., resistance to change, peculiar interest in or attachments to animate or inanimate objects.
6. Absence of delusions, hallucinations, loosening of associations, and incoherence as in schizophrenia.

[a]American Psychiatric Association. (1980). *Diagnostic and statistical manual of mental disorders* (3rd ed.). Washington, DC: Author.

Owing to the early onset of symptoms, pharmacotherapy may be initiated during the early childhood period. Unfortunately, few of the drugs that are effective for the treatment of infantile autism are approved for use with children under the age of 6 years. A detailed discussion of this topic is presented in the following section. Ironically, many more well-controlled medication studies appear to have been conducted on preschool-aged autistic children than on any other age group.

Hypnotics and anticonvulsants are of no value in the treatment of childhood psychosis, and barbiturates may only aggravate the disorder. Stimulants (Benzedrine, Dexedrine, Ritalin) are *generally* not effective even if hyperactivity is a prominent problem. Often, these drugs make the psychotic symptoms even worse by decreasing verbal output and making the child more withdrawn. In general, the tricyclic antidepressants (e.g., Tofranil) have not proved to be effective (they may make things even worse) nor have the hallucinogens (e.g., LSD–25).

Few agents have proved really helpful for psychotic children. Benadryl, an antihistamine with sedative properties, has been administered with some success in severely disturbed children (Fish, 1971). The neuroleptics, however, are the most useful and most frequently prescribed drugs for childhood psychosis. The phenothiazines (Thorazine, Mellaril, Stelazine) have been quite effective with school-aged and adolescent schizophrenic children but are less desirable for young children because their associated side effects may have special implications for later development. Neuroleptics that are more "stimulating" (e.g., Haldol and Navane) are generally more preferred. When neuroleptic medication works, the therapeutic response takes the form of increased responsiveness and alertness and a brightening of mood. Some children are described as more talkative and less withdrawn. Suppression of undesirable behaviors such as stereotypy, hyperactivity, aggressivity, and self-injury are also reported.

Dosage guidelines for the neuroleptics are difficult to set down because there is a great deal of variability across children. Titration is the recommended procedure, and the optimal dose in mg/kg may be higher than for adults. This may be explained, in part, by the fact that children metabolize many types of drugs at a faster rate than adults.

The side effects of the neuroleptics must be monitored quite carefully. Even though the incidence of extrapyramidal syndromes appears to be low in autistic children, suppression of adaptive behavior is always a possibility. In this regard, Campbell (1975) stated that:

> The young child is often excessively sedated at doses that control certain psychotic symptoms. In our experience, many of these children show sleepiness and psychomotor retardation even at very low doses of chlorpromazine (Thorazine) and are not amenable to education and other treatment, irrespective of body weight and the presence or absence of hyperactivity and aggressiveness. (pp. 240–241)

Several additional comments are in order about drug management. First, children who respond favorably to one type of drug at an early age may do much better on a different medication when older. Also, the search for an effective agent may be a long and tedious process of gradually adjusting the dose and assessing therapeutic benefits. It may also require trials of several different drugs. Second, the duration of treatment varies depending upon the magnitude of the therapeutic response, which should be evaluated at periodic intervals. Finally, relatively little is known about the use of neuroleptics with young children; therefore, careful monitoring is in order. Drug-free periods should be scheduled regularly to assess the continued need for treatment (Fish, 1976).

> Once a child's development has been stimulated by using medication, and his speech or other performance has become established, these gains may continue without further medication. One does not want to introduce substances into the body unless they are really necessary. (p. 114)

One of the newest drugs for the treatment of autism is Pondimin (fenfluramine). It is approved by the Food and Drug Administration (FDA) in the United States for the treatment of obesity and is pharmacologically similar to the amphetamines (e.g., Dexedrine). The drug appears to decrease hyperactivity and distractibility and possibly increases intellectual ability (Ritvo et al., 1983). The daily dose employed in one study with children was 1.5 mg/kg per day, which was divided into a morning and an afternoon dose (August et al., 1985). Side effects were mild and included weight loss and lethargy. Many children appear to experience a rebound effect (irritability, restlessness, aggressivity) upon drug withdrawal.

Drug Therapy: Early Childhood

Much of our knowledge about the use of pharmacotherapy in the management of autism in preschool-aged children stems from the research efforts of Barbara Fish and more recently Magda Campbell at Bellevue Hospital in New York City. There are additional psychotropic drug studies with elementary school–aged youngsters that do include 4 and 5 year olds, particularly in the case of more severely handicapping conditions, but they are rarely treated as a separate subgroup for data analysis.

Most of the well-controlled neuroleptic drug studies with preschool-aged children are listed in Table 4–3 by the trade name of the drug under investigation. Drug dosages are also presented, but it must be realized that with the exception of Mellaril, Thorazine, and Haldol, none of the agents are approved by the FDA for use with children under 6 years as of this writing. Dosages for Mellaril and Thorazine reported in the *Physicians' Desk Reference* (1985) are as follows: For Mellaril, the dose for children between 2 and 12 years ranges from 0.5 mg/kg per day to 3.0 mg/kg per day. For Thorazine, the dosage for child outpatients with a psychiatric disorder is 0.25 mg per *pound* administered every 4 to 6 hours.

In autistic children, neuroleptic drugs reduce withdrawal, hyperactivity, stereotypies, fidgetiness, and abnormal object relations. Haldol is superior to the phenothiazines (e.g., Thorazine) because it is less likely to cause sedation at optimal dosages. Haldol has also been shown to increase the effectiveness of a language-based behavior therapy program (Campbell et al., 1978) and appears to facilitate discrimination learning (Anderson et al., 1984). The *optimal* dose for most preschoolers ranges between 0.5 to 1.0 mg per day. *Hypoactive* autistic children are not helped by treatment with Haldol, and their symptoms may even become worse.

The duration of treatment is determined, in part, by the degree to which the drug continues to produce a clinically meaningful therapeutic response. This can only be assessed with systematic dosage reductions and drug-free periods. One study has shown that Haldol remained clinically effective even after 2½ years (Campbell et al., 1983). Nevertheless, other children in that same investigation no longer required drug therapy after several months of medication.

Table 4–3. Reported Antipsychotic Oral Drug Dosages for Preschool-Aged Children

Drug	Study	Age (years)	Disorder	Dose (mg/day)	Dose (mean)
Haldol (haloperidol)	Campbell et al. (1978)	2.6–7.2	Infantile autism	0.5–4.0	1.65
	Cohen et al. (1980)	2.1–7.0	Infantile autism	0.5–4.0	1.78
	Anderson et al. (1984)	2.3–6.9	Infantile autism	0.5–3.0	1.11
Lithium carbonate	Campbell et al. (1972)	3.0–6.0	Infantile autism	450–900	735
Moban (molindone)	Campbell et al. (1971)	3–5	Infantile autism	1–2.5	1.5
Navane (thiothixene)	Campbell et al. (1970)	3–5	Infantile autism	1–6	2.0
Stelazine (trifluoperazine)	Fish et al. (1966)	2–6	Infantile autism	2–20	8.2
	Fish et al. (1969)	2–5	Infantile autism	2–8	4
Thorazine (chlorpromazine)	Fish et al. (1969)	2–5	Infantile autism	30–150	75
	Campbell et al. (1972)	3–6	Infantile autism	9–45	17.3

Dosage adjustment is a critical procedure anytime therapy involves a drug whose intended effect is the facilitation of adaptive behavior. Because young autistic children typically receive special education and other services, medication should be used only when it leads to more rapid cognitive, academic, or social development. The following is a description of dosage adjustment procedures and the management of untoward drug reactions by Campbell et al. (1984a):

> Dosage regulation in children requires daily observations performed in a variety of different settings with the close cooperation of the physician, parents, and teachers. Dosage regulation is also difficult because optimal dosage can differ between children of the same approximate size, weight, and body surface area. In most instances, dosage regulation can be more easily performed in an inpatient setting. After an adequate period of baseline assessment, drug therapy should begin with the administration of low, often therapeutically ineffective doses. The baseline assessment should include the identification of target symptoms (e.g., aggressiveness, hyperactivity, stereotypies, withdrawal) and careful recording of any involuntary movements (frequency and topography). Dosage increments should be gradual and made on a regular basis no more frequently than twice weekly. The major therapeutic task is to avoid excessive sedation at doses which attenuate target symptoms: Polypharmacy in children is to be avoided.
>
> The emergence of untoward effects may necessitate dosage reduction. Unlike in adults, affectomotor side effects (e.g., irritability, alterations in level of motor activity) occur commonly with neuroleptic administration to children. On the other hand, parkinsonian side effects appear to be a function of age: the younger the child, the less frequent their occurrence. These side effects in children are best treated by dosage reduction. Antiparkinsonian medication is avoided because there is some evidence that they may reduce serum neuroleptic levels (Rivera-Calimlim et al., 1976) and contribute to worsening of behavioral symptoms and cognition due to central anticholinergic properties. Acute dystonic reactions are less frequent if drug is begun with very low doses and increases are gradual. However, should they occur, they are usually rapidly responsive to diphenhydramine (Benadryl), either orally or intramuscularly (25 mg). These dystonic reactions result from involuntary contractions of skeletal muscle groups and may be manifest as painful stiffening or arching of the back, neck, or tongue, and oculogyric crisis. (pp. 112–113)

In addition to acute dystonic reaction, preschoolers are at risk for the development of other extrapyramidal symptoms as well. One long-term treatment study of Haldol found that 22% of the children developed *dyskinesias* (like those associated with tardive dyskinesia) either during treatment or when switched to placebo. In a few cases the dyskinesias were manifested as an aggravation of preexisting stereotypies. The dyskinesias appeared anywhere from 5 weeks to 16 months after the onset of treatment. The dyskinesias stopped within 16 days to 9 months after they first began. In some cases they ceased while the child was on medication, and in others after they had been switched to a placebo or medication was discontinued.

Megavitamins

After reviewing the literature, the American Academy of Pediatrics (1976) reported that megavitamins were of little value in the treatment of childhood psychosis. Recently, however, a well-controlled study demonstrated that a small percentage of autistic children might benefit from such treatment (Rimland et al., 1978). Sixteen autistic children who appeared to improve in a previous study when receiving vitamin B_6 (pyridoxine) were selected for a B_6 and placebo comparison. The investigators reported a deterioration in symptoms for 11 of the children when placed on placebo. The dose of B_6 ranged from 2.4 to 94.3 mg/kg per day; median dose was approximately 6 mg/kg per day.

There is a general air of suspicion among scientists concerning megavitamin therapy, primarily because its touted benefits for a host of disorders are not based upon empirical fact and are greatly exaggerated. This is an unfortunate but very typical phenomenon in medicine and generally occurs in the early stages of discovery and confirmation of clinical utility. The problems with this therapeutic approach are threefold: (a) response appears to be idiosyncratic and next to impossible to predict; (b) because there are so many different substances associated with this approach, discovering the right ingredient (or combination of ingredients) may take some time; and (c) at certain dosages, some vitamins can be lethal or cause serious adverse reactions. Given this situation, it is imperative that efficacy be objectively established on a case-by-case basis. In other words, either behavior rating scales, direct observations, or performance tests should be used every time this treatment is prescribed.

Nondrug Therapies

Autistic children require intense educational intervention to facilitate the acquisition of language and social skills and to suppress maladaptive behaviors (see Rutter, 1985, for a recent review). There exists a truly impressive literature on the effectiveness of behavior therapy techniques with this population, and they are routinely employed in exemplary intervention programs. As was previously noted, drug researchers have been emphatic about the *adjunctive* role of medication in the treatment of autistic children and adolescents. Although there are some data to suggest that neuroleptic medication may make educational interventions more effective (Campbell et al., 1978), the magnitude of the therapeutic benefit from medication is in general modest. In short, even on medication these children remain seriously handicapped.

CONDUCT DISORDER, AGGRESSIVE

Conduct disorder refers to a persistent pattern of antisocial behavior. A distinction is made between conduct-disordered children who are socialized (have friends but are manipulative of others and show a lack of concern for those outside of their own clique) and undersocialized (generally do not have true friends or show feelings of guilt or remorse and exploit others for self-gain). A distinction is also made between aggressive and nonaggressive subtypes. The aggressive subtype is characterized by "physical violence against persons" or "thefts outside the home involving confrontation with a victim" (American Psychiatric Association, 1980). Stated examples of these behaviors include mugging, assault, homicide, and extortion. Because few prepubertal children engage in rape or armed robbery, it will be difficult for some to see the relevance of this disorder for the elementary school age group. When confronted with this apparent oversight, clinicians may state that these are only examples of antisocial behavior and appropriate ones can be easily generated for the younger child (e.g., fighting with classmates). Nevertheless, it is still unclear exactly what is meant when an investigator states that his or her study employed prepubertal children diagnosed as conduct disorder, undersocialized, aggressive. The diagnostic criteria for this condition appear in Table 4–4. For a diagnosis of conduct disorder, socialized, aggressive, item No. 2 should read: "evidence of social attachment to others as indicated by at least two of the following behavior patterns" (p. 49).

There is another condition, conduct disorder, nonaggressive, which is based on any one of the following symptoms (American Psychiatric Association, 1980):

1. chronic violations of a variety of important rules (that are reasonable and age-appropriate for the child) at home or at school (e.g., persistent truancy, substance abuse)
2. repeated running away from home overnight
3. persistent serious lying in and out of the home
4. stealing not involving confrontation with a victim. (p. 49)

Because medication is generally not prescribed for such things as a persistent pattern of lying, stealing, or running away, this disorder is

Table 4–4. DSM III Diagnostic Criteria for Conduct Disorder, Undersocialized, Aggressive*

---

1. A receptive and persistent pattern of aggressive conduct in which the basic rights of others are violated, as manifested by either of the following:

    (a) physical violence against persons or property (not to defend someone else or oneself), e.g., vandalism, rape, breaking and entering, fire-setting, mugging, assault
    (a) thefts outside the home involving confrontation with the victim (e.g., extortion, purse-snatching, armed robbery)

2. Failure to establish a normal degree of affection, empathy, or bond with others as evidenced by *no more than one* of the following indications of social attachment:

    (a) has one or more peer-group friendships that have lasted over six months
    (b) extends himself or herself for others even when no immediate advantage is likely
    (c) apparently feels guilt or remorse when such a reaction is appropriate (not just when caught or in difficulty)
    (d) avoids blaming or informing on companions
    (e) shares concern for the welfare of friends or companions

3. Duration of pattern of aggressive conduct of at least six months.

4. If 18 or older, does not meet the criteria for Antisocial Personality Disorder.

---

*American Psychiatric Association. (1980). *Diagnostic and statistical manual of mental disorders* (3rd ed). Washington, DC: Author.

not addressed here. It is, of course, possible that these behaviors may be exhibited in children and adolescents who suffer from some other type of psychiatric disorder for which psychotropic drugs may be prescribed.

There are no data on the prevalence of conduct disorder, aggressive, as it is defined in DSM III or on the extent of drug therapy for it. Lest this statement be misinterpreted, it should be noted that conduct disorders, more broadly defined as "fighting and other forms of aggression, disobedience, destructiveness, and meanness" have been studied systematically for at least two decades (see Stewart et al., 1980). Children who are diagnosed as being hyperactive (attention deficit disorder with hyperactivity) are often aggressive, particularly those who are referred to child psychiatry clinics (see Loney & Millich, 1982), and many are subsequently treated with stimulant medication. When a hyperactive child is severely aggressive, the clinician is more inclined to try a neuroleptic drug, especially in cases when stimulant medication is only marginally effective. However, neuroleptic drugs when used at clinically effective doses are often associated with side effects that can impair adaptive behavior in the classroom. Therefore, there is an intense interest in discovering more suitable drugs for the treatment of aggressive behavior.

Drug Therapy

In their review of the literature on the effectiveness of drug therapy for aggressive behavior, Campbell et al. (1982) noted the need for more well-controlled studies in this area. They also presented the results of a pilot study that included a subsample of prepubertal children who met the diagnostic criteria for conduct disorder, undersocialized. aggressive. It was found that while Thorazine produced excessive sedation at therapeutic doses (100 to 200 mg per day or 2.8 mg/kg to 5.8 mg/kg per day), Haldol was much more well tolerated (4 to 16 mg per day or 0.12 to 0.75 mg/kg per day).

The pilot study was followed by a thorough and well-controlled investigation into the effects of Haldol and lithium carbonate on hospitalized conduct-disordered, undersocialized, aggressive children between 5 and 13 years old (Campbell et al., 1984c). The optimum dosage of Haldol ranged from 1.0 to 6.0 mg per day (0.04 to 0.21 mg/kg per day), and the optimum dose of lithium was 500 to 2,000 mg per day (or serum levels of 0.32 to 1.51 mEq/L). Both Haldol and lithium were highly effective in reducing aggressive behavior (see Figure 4-1). Qualitatively, whereas Haldol rendered the children more manageable, lithium reduced the explosive nature of their aggressive behavior, which enabled other positive changes to take place. Subjectively, the children on Haldol felt "slowed down" and the youngsters receiving lithium thought that medication "helped to control" themselves. The most common side effects of Haldol were excessive sedation (e.g., drowsiness), acute dystonic reaction, and drooling. The acute dystonic reaction was relieved with a single 25 mg dose of Benadryl administered orally or intramuscularly. The emergence of acute dystonic reactions can often be avoided by using a small starting dose (e.g., 0.5 mg) and making dose increments on a gradual and protracted schedule. Adverse reactions to lithium included stomachache, headache, and tremor of the hands. It appeared that the optimal dose of Haldol interfered with daily functioning more than lithium (Figure 4-2).

The use of lithium for the treatment of childhood disorders (see Campbell et al., 1984b, for a review) is becoming a more widely accepted practice. There are, therefore, several additional comments that should be made regarding this agent. One, the appropriate use of lithium requires periodic venipuncture (drawing of blood) to determine blood levels and subsequently ensure that the child is not in the toxic range. This will be difficult with uncooperative children

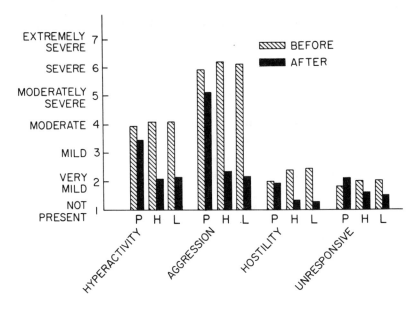

Figure 4–1. Child psychiatrists' mean ratings on four clusters of items from the Children's Psychiatric Rating Scale, before (baseline) and at the end of 6 weeks of treatment (sixth week) for three treatment groups: Placebo (P), Haldol (H), and Lithium (L). From "Behavioral Efficacy of Haloperidol and Lithium Carbonate" by M. Campbell et al., 1984c. *Archives of General Psychiatry, 41,* p. 652. Copyright 1984 by the American Medical Association. Adapted by permission.

and is probably best done in an inpatient setting, at least while dosage is being titrated to determine the optimal level. Unfortunately, analysis of saliva drug levels does not appear to be a suitable substitute for blood analysis (Perry et al., 1984). Two, lithium is not recommended for children under 12 years of age by the FDA in the United States because there is insufficient research on this age group. Three, lithium is contraindicated for patients with kidney, liver, heart, or thyroid disease. Moreover, there is a risk of birth defects associated with lithium treatment, so it should be used with caution for teenage girls who may become pregnant. Four, adequate salt and fluid intake is required to prevent toxic levels from developing in the blood. This is particularly important during warm weather, which may lead to fluid loss from sweating. Lastly, lithium does not appear to have an adverse effect on cognition at optimum dosages (Platt et al., 1984). The same unfortunately cannot be said for Haldol.

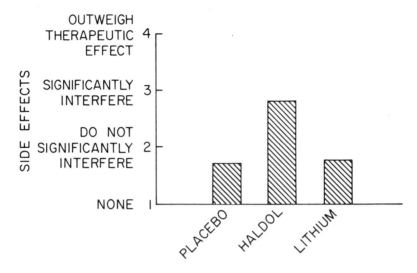

Figure 4–2. Child psychiatrists' mean ratings of side effects with optimal dosage on Clinical Global impressions scale. From "Behavioral Efficacy of Haloperidol and Lithium Carbonate" by M. Campbell et al., 1984c. *Archives of General Psychiatry, 41,* p. 653. Copyright 1984 by the American Medical Association. Adapted by permission.

Another drug that may be helpful for the treatment of severe aggression and explosive fits of rage is Inderal (propranolol). Dosage and side effects information are presented in Chapter 5. Its use for the treatment of conduct-disordered, undersocialized, aggressive children and adolescents is based upon the findings from one uncontrolled study (Williams et al., 1982). The following case study from Williams et al. is an excellent example of the type of child for which purported claims of efficacy have been made:

Tom, a 13½-year-old 8th grade public school student, was admitted . . . because of episodic rage outbursts since the first year of life. Tom . . . had pneumonia with high fever during the first week home, [and] . . . subsequently, he was very cranky, with severe head banging at 9 months of age, as well as implacable crying and screaming. Persistent behavioral problems at age 2 prompted an EEG, which was reportedly abnormal. Tom was given Dilantin and phenobarbital, which initially seemed to help calm him somewhat. . . .At age 3 he fell down a flight of stairs, striking his head. This was followed by an apparent seizure . . . He was thereafter maintained on anticonvulsants without any further clinical seizures. Yet his behavior over the years continued to be characterized by aggressiveness and explosiveness that including cursing, screaming, running away, suicidal threats as well as fights with classmates and siblings. When restricted to his room, he had punched holes in the walls and door with his fist or a knife and had destroyed all the furniture in his room. There was no family history of seizures or of major psychiatric illness. Multiple psychiatric consultations, including trials on various analeptics and neuroleptics, were uniformly unsuccessful.

Psychiatric interview with Tom on admission disclosed him to be an alert, articulate and cooperative boy, who manifested no thought disorder, no inappropriate affect and no bizarre behavior. His mood was sad in describing his outbursts and he seemed resigned to being "sent away to boarding school," which was the then current plan, "because my family can't handle me." EEG on this admission. . . . was normal . . . Psychological testing disclosed an. . . . IQ of 102, but Tom's reading, spelling and arithmetic scores on the WRAT were all 2 years behind grade level. . . . A conjoint decision was made . . . to taper Tom off Dilantin, the only medication he was then taking, and concomitantly start propranolol, 10 mg p.o. 4 times a day, to be titrated upward by the patient's treating psychiatrist. At a dose of 40 mg p.o. 4 times a day, Tom's parents noted marked and sustained improvement in his behavior. Plans for boarding school were dropped, but special educational help was provided. Occasional supportive psychotherapy sessions monitored Tom's status, which continued stable over the course of 16 months despite serious marital strife between his parents. Three attempts to taper the propranolol during this time resulted in behavioral relapses, prompting its reinstitution. A fourth trial, initiated by Tom's disinclination to take the medication, resulted in a satisfactory state of behavioral control free of rage outbursts over the subsequent 6 months with no concomitant psychotherapy. (p. 133)

DEPRESSION (CHILDHOOD)

A great deal of interest has been generated over the existence of depression in prepubertal children (Conners, 1976; Rapoport, 1976), and most of the research on this disorder has appeared within the last decade. Once considered a very rare condition (Graham, 1974; Rutter et al., 1970), more recent surveys show that the prevalence of *major depressive disorder* in prepubertal children in the United States and in New Zealand is approximately 1.8% (Kashani & Simonds, 1979; Kashani et al., 1983). One study found that teachers appeared to be less aware of depressive symptoms than parents and that the behavior of depressed children did not differ from normal controls during psychological testing (Kashani et al, 1983). Moreover, many of the children who fit the criteria for depression are not taken for psychological or psychiatric help (Kashani et al., 1983; Kovacs et al., 1984), and few are currently treated with medication (Kovacs et al., 1984). Therefore, at the present time, it is accurate to say that the prevalence of drug treatment for childhood depression must be extremely low. Children with major depressive disorder are unlikely to recover within the first 3 months of the depressive episode, but remission generally occurs 6 to 18 months (92%) (Kovacs et al., 1984). If the child does not recover by that time, the illness is likely to be protracted. The more early the age of onset of the disorder the longer the recovery period.

The symptoms upon which a diagnosis of major depressive disorder in childhood is based are the same as those for adults according to DSM III (American Psychiatric Association, 1980). They are presented in Table 4–5.

Children who meet the diagnostic criteria for major depressive disorder may also experience other psychiatric problems as well. Many have conduct disorders (Carlson & Cantwell, 1980; Puig-Antich, 1982) or exhibit antisocial behavior (Geller et al., 1985), anxiety disorder (Kovacs et al., 1984), separation anxiety (Geller et al., 1985), school phobia (Kolvin et al., 1984), or psychotic symptoms such as hallucinations or delusions (Freeman et al., 1985). A good example of a "mixed" presentation with psychotic symptoms is provided in a case study from Freeman et al. (1985):

> His developmental history was unremarkable except that he had allergies and frequent upper respiratory infections. His parents said Buddy was a "normal, healthy" child until 8 months prior to evaluation. He then began to complain of severe stomach and chest pains. . . . His complaints and his frequent emergency room visits persisted and increased 2 months prior to evaluation. At that time, his maternal grandmother died after a myocardial infarction.
>
> After her death, his other symptoms began to appear. Buddy began to excessively wash his hands. He had difficulty going to sleep and began to sleep with his mother (his father worked the night shift). His classmates began to "pick on him" and he was frequently in fights at school. In one altercation, he hit a boy with his lunch box, cutting the child's head so that the wound required several sutures. One month prior to evaluation, Buddy began to refuse to go to school.
>
> At the evaluation, Buddy appeared tense, anxious, and agitated. His affect was moderately restricted and worried. He spoke in a pressured manner about his "problems." Buddy had been feeling "sad and bored" several hours a day. He described irritability and agitation. His concentration was poor "I can't read—I can't pay attention." He was afraid of dying—"I might get stabbed or shot." He felt guilty and down on himself. He described auditory hallucinations like hearing "people say 'your grandmother says she loves you,' " or a voice saying "kill someone." He had heard his grandmother's voice saying "I hope you feel better" and "I will always love you." God told him, "Don't eat." Buddy was convinced his food was poisoned and refused to eat. He said "the reason I'm stick is because someone put poison in my body." He thought that "someone wants to hurt me, I can tell because the lights go on and off in my house."

Table 4–5.   DSM III Criteria for a Diagnosis for Major Depressive Episode[a]

---

1. Dysphoric mood or loss of interest or pleasure in all or almost all usual activities and pastimes. The dysphoric mood is characterized by symptoms such as the following: depressed, sad, blue, hopeless, low, down in the dumps, irritable. The mood disturbance must be prominent and relatively persistent, but not necessarily the most dominant symptom, and does not include momentary shifts from one dysphoric mood to another dysphoric mood, e.g., anxiety to depression to anger, such as are seen in states of acute psychotic turmoil. (For children under six, dysphoric mood may have to be inferred from a persistently sad facial expression.)

2. At least four of the following symptoms have each been present nearly every day for a period of at least two weeks (in children under six, at least three of the first four).

    (a) poor appetite or significant weight loss (when not dieting) or increased appetite or significant weight gain (in children under six, consider failure to make expected weight gains)
    (b) insomnia or hypersomnia
    (c) psychomotor agitation or retardation (but not merely subjective feelings of restlessness or being slowed down) (in children under six, hypoactivity)
    (d) loss of interest or pleasure in usual activities, or decrease in sexual drive not limited to a period when delusional or hallucinating (in children under six, signs of apathy)
    (e) loss of energy; fatigue
    (f) feelings of worthlessness, self-reproach, or excessive or inappropriate guilt (either may be delusional)
    (g) complaints or evidence of diminished ability to think or concentrate, such as slowed thinking, or indecisiveness not associated with marked loosening of associations or incoherence.
    (h) recurrent thoughts of death, suicidal ideation, wishes to be dead, or suicide attempt

3. Neither of the following dominate the clinical picture when an affective syndrome (i.e., criteria 1 and 2 above) is not present, that is, before it developed or after it has remitted:

    (a) preoccupation with a mood-incongruent delusion or hallucination (see definition below)
    (b) bizarre behavior

4. Not superimposed on either Schizophrenia, Schizophreniform Disorder, or a Paranoid Disorder.

5. Not due to any Organic Mental Disorder or Uncomplicated Bereavement.

---

[a]American Psychiatric Association. (1980). *Diagnostic and statistical manual of mental disorders* (3rd ed.). Washington, DC: Author

The family history revealed his mother had a dysthymic disorder after Buddy's birth. His father had alcohol abuse and dysthymic disorder.

Buddy was admitted to a children's inpatient unit for 21 days of observation and treatment. He was noted to be anxious, reclusive, fearful, avoiding other children, and needing the constant attention of adults. He was treated with desipramine and discharged to his parents' care. Outpatient family therapy was prescribed. At 6 weeks after evaluation, Buddy was no longer depressed. Although he sometimes worried his food might be poisoned, he was no longer convinced of this and ate regularly. He had no hallucinations. (p. 99)

Drug Therapy

There are now a number of reports on the use of tricyclic antidepressants for the treatment of major depressive disorder in children, a few of which are noted here. Tofranil (imipramine) has been used to treat this condition (Petti & Law, 1982; Puig-Antich, 1982; Puig-Antich et al., 1979), with dosages of 5 mg/kg per day or higher if necessary (Puig-Antich, 1982). Children who did not tolerate higher doses of Tofranil were given desmethylimipramine (not approved for general use in the United States). Elavil (amitriptyline) at a dosage of 1.5 mg/kg per day (45 to 110 mg) may be effective in improving mood and level of interest as evidenced by a greater desire to play with other children and purportedly is associated with few side effects (Kashani et al., 1984). Other tricyclics that have been studied or reported on with use for depressed children are Aventyl (nortriptyline) and Norpramin or Pertofrane (desipramine) (Freeman et al., 1985; Geller et al., 1984). Depressed children who respond best to these medications are more likely to have higher concentrations of the drug in their blood (regardless of dose) and family members who have a history of depressive illness.

SCHIZOPHRENIA (CHILDHOOD)

Many clinicians make a distinction between childhood *schizophrenia* and (early) infantile autism (e.g., Rutter, 1972). Nevertheless, a considerable degree of controversy does and has existed over the existence of this disorder. Childhood schizophrenia now generally refers to prepubertal children who exhibit the symptoms of schizophrenia. In other words, according to the American Psychiatric Association (1980), the diagnostic criteria for adult, adolescent, and child schizophrenia are the same (see Table 5–2, Adolescent Disorders). Although a table of symptoms does give some idea of what the disorder is like, for someone who has not worked with these children it is difficult to appreciate how such a child might behave. The following case description of an 8-year-old schizophrenic boy (who had a history of earlier schizophrenic episode at the age of 5 years) prepared by Green et al. (1984) provides a graphic illustration of this disorder:

The child came from a wealthy middle class family, of concerned parents. As an infant he seldom smiled and did not like to be cuddled. He was a fearful toddler and exhibited sibling rivalry. After a bilingual nursery he entered kindergarten at the age of 5 years. A month later he suddenly developed hallucinations and delusions. He became fearful of insects which were "all over his body," of electricity (believed his parents and doctors might get electrocuted) and expressed concern about eating too much food and about passing insects with his bowel movements. He had a complete neurological workup which was normal. He was treated with chlorpromazine and discharged 5 days after admission, with marked improvement. He continued with chemotherapy and individual and family therapy for 10 more months. In school he appeared to be sad and withdrawn. He got into frequent fights with peers. Academic work was satisfactory, while in arts and other less structured activities he would become distractible, volatile and inappropriate. At the age of 8, after some slight school difficulty with a peer who scratched him on his forehead, the patient became increasingly anxious, unable to function in school, developed auditory and visual hallucinations, somatic delusions, and paranoid ideation. He was afraid that people in his house wanted to kill him and his younger brother. He was spitting and yelling all the time. He used neologisms both in English and Chinese. He complained of his body being "invaded" by devils; he heard God's voice and saw devils' faces on his blanket. His symptoms increased and he required hospitalization because of failure to respond to outpatient treatment including thioridazine. On admission he was agitated and walked like an automaton. His speech was disconnected and he kept asking "Who am I. . . . am I Peter. . . . am I John. . . . who am I. . . . At times he was catatonic. Hallucinations and delusions failed to respond to a variety of treatments which included haloperidol. Though his hospital course fluctuated, this seemed to have no relationship to treatment. (pp. 406–407)

Childhood schizophrenia is a rare disorder, and it does appear to be a separate diagnostic entity from infantile autism. Moreover, children with infantile autism do not become indistinguishable from schizophrenics during the elementary school years (Green et al., 1984). One important difference between the two groups reported in Green et al.'s study is that none of the autistic children had hallucinations or delusions on clinical examination, but most of the schizophrenic children experienced auditory (79%) or visual (46%) hallucinations or delusions (54%).

Hallucinations are an uncommon phenomenon in children. Prevalence figures range from ½ to 1%. One study of childhood psychiatric patients identified 25 children who experienced true hallucinations but who were not necessarily schizophrenic (Burke et al., 1985). One half had auditory hallucinations only, and the other half experienced both auditory and visual hallucinations. The auditory hallucinations consisted of voices talking to the child, voices telling the child to hurt others, or mumbling. The following are some examples from Burke et al.:

> (a) an 8-year-old boy reported hearing voices telling him to stab his sister, to stab a playmate, and to poke needles in his 2-year-old sister's eyes; (b) a 12-year-old boy heard a voice calling his name and a second voice which talked to him in a frightening way; (c) an 8-year-old boy heard a man's voice and a woman's voice, one telling him to hurt children and one telling him not to; (d) an 11-year-old boy heard voices yelling and saying they would hurt him; (e) an 11-year-old boy heard voices telling him to kill himself and to be destructive; and (f) a 9-year-old boy heard indistinct mumbling voices. (p. 72)

Interestingly, with the exception of the children who were diagnosed as having clear psychotic episodes, the hallucinations were a long-standing phenomenon for these children.

The prognosis for children with childhood schizophrenia is not good (Eggers, 1978) but may be better than what was previously thought (Kydd & Werry, 1982). Improvement at followup was reported at 50% by Eggers, but *remission* (marked decrease in or cessation of symptoms) was limited to 20 to 40% (Eggers, 1978; Kydd & Werry, 1982).

Childhood schizophrenia is generally treated with neuroleptic medication. Because pharmacotherapy for adolescent schizophrenia is discussed in Chapter 5 (Adolescent Disorders), it is not repeated here. Moreover, the preceding discussion of pharmacotherapy for autism (infantile) has direct application to childhood schizophrenia. Neuroleptic drug dosages for children under 12 years of age appear in Table 4–1.

SUGGESTED READINGS

Campbell, M., Anderson, L. T., Deutsch, S. I., & Green, W. H. (1984a). Psychopharmacological treatment of children with the syndrome of autism. *Pediatric Annals, 13,* 309–316. (C,S)

Campbell, M., Cohen, I. L., & Anderson, L. T. (1981). Pharmacotherapy for autistic children: A summary of research. *Canadian Journal of Psychiatry, 26,* 265–273. (C,S)

Campbell, M., & Deutsch, S. I. (1985). Neuroleptics in children. In G. D. Burrows, T. Norman, & B. Davies (Ed.), *Drugs in Psychiatry (Vol. 3): Antipsychotics* (pp. 213–238). New York: Elsevier Biomedical. (C)

Campbell, M., Perry, R., & Green, W. H. (1984b). Use of lithium in children and adolescents. *Psychosomatics, 25,* 95–106. (C)

Rutter, M. (1985). The treatment of autistic children. *Journal of Child Psychology and Psychiatry, 26,* 193–214. (C,S)

REFERENCES

Algozzine, B. (1977). The emotionally disturbed child: Disturbed or disturbing. *Journal of Abnormal Child Psychology, 5,* 205–211.

Aman, M. G. (1984). Drugs and learning in mentally retarded persons. In G. D. Burrows & J. S. Werry (Eds.), *Advances in human psychopharmacology* (Vol. 3, pp. 121–163). Greenwich, CT: JAI Press.

Aman, M. G. & Singh, N. N. (1983). Pharmacological intervention. In J. L. Matson & J. A. Mulick (Eds.), *Handbook of mental retardation* (pp. 317–337). New York: Pergamon.

American Academy of Pediatrics. (1976). Megavitamin therapy for childhood psychoses and learning disabilities. *Pediatrics, 58,* 910–912.

American Psychiatric Association. (1980). *Diagnostic and statistical manual of mental disorders* (3rd ed.). Washington, DC: Author.

Anderson, L. T., Campbell, M., Grega, D. M., Perry, R., Small, A. M., & Green, W. H. (1984). Haloperidol in the treatment of infantile autism: Effects on learning and behavioral symptoms. *American Journal of Psychiatry, 141,* 1195–1202.

August, G. J., Raz, N., & Baird, T. D. (1985). Brief report: Effects of fenfluramine on behavioral, cognitive, and affective disturbances in autistic children. *Journal of Autism and Developmental Disorders, 15,* 97–107.

Baldessarini, R. J. (1980). Drugs and the treatment of psychiatric disorders. In A. G. Gilman, L. S. Goodman, & A. Gilman (Eds.), *The pharmacological basis of therapeutics* (6th ed., pp. 391–447). New York: Macmillan.

Bender, L., & Nichtern, S. (1956). Chemotherapy in child psychiatry. *New York State Journal of Medicine, 56,* 2791–2795.

Bradley, C. (1958). Tranquilizing drugs in pediatrics. *Pediatrics, 21,* 325–300.

Bricklin, P. M., & Gallico, R. (1984). Learning disabilities and emotional disturbance: Critical issues in definition, assessment, and service delivery. *Learning Disabilities, 3,* 141–156.

Burke, P., DelBeccaro, M., McCauley, E., & Clark, C. (1985). Hallucinations in children. *Journal of the American Academy of Child Psychiatry, 24,* 71–75.

Campbell, M. (1975). Psychopharmacology in childhood psychosis. *International Journal of Mental Health, 4,* 238–254.

Campbell, M., Anderson, L. T., Deutsch, S. I., & Green, W. H. (1984a). Psychopharmacological treatment of children with the syndrome of autism. *Pediatric Annals, 13,* 309–316.

Campbell, M., Anderson, L. T., Meier, M., Cohen, I. L., Small, A. M., Samit, C., & Sachar, E. J. (1978). A comparison of haloperidol and behavior therapy and their interaction in autistic children. *Journal of the American Academy of Child Psychiatry, 17,* 640–655.

Campbell, M., Cohen, I. L., & Anderson, L. T. (1981). Pharmacotherapy for autistic children: A summary of research. *Canadian Journal of Psychiatry, 26,* 265–273.

Campbell, M., Cohen, I. L., & Small, A. M. (1982). Drugs and aggressive behavior. *Journal of the American Academy of Child Psychiatry, 21,* 107–117.

Campbell, M., & Deutsch, S. I. (1985). Neuroleptics in children. In G. D. Burrows, T. Norman, & B. Davies (Eds.), *Drugs in psychiatry (Vol. 3): Antipsychotics* (pp. 213–238). New York: Elsevier Biomedical.

Campbell, M., Fish, B., Korein, J., Shapiro, T., Collins, P., & Koh, C. (1972). Lithium and chlorpromazine: A controlled cross-over study of hyperactive severely disturbed young children. *Journal of Autism and Childhood Schizophrenia, 2,* 234–263.

Campbell, M., Fish, B., Shapiro, T., & Floyd, A., Jr. (1970). Thiothixene in young disturbed children: A pilot study. *Archives of General Psychiatry, 23,* 70–72.

Campbell, M., Fish, B., Shapiro, T., Floyd, A., Jr. (1971). Study of molindone in disturbed preschool children. *Current Therapeutic Research, 13,* 28–33.

Campbell, M., Perry, R., Bennett, W. G., Small, A. M., Green, W. H., Grega, D., Schwartz, V., & Anderson, L. (1983). Long-term therapeutic efficacy and drug-related abnormal movements: A prospective study of haloperidol in autistic children. *Psychopharmacology Bulletin, 19,* 80–83.

Campbell, M., Perry, R., & Green, W. H. (1984b). Use of lithium in children and adolescents. *Psychosomatics, 2,* 95–106.

Campbell, M., Small, A. M., Green, W. H., Jennings, S. J., Perry, R., Bennett, W. G., & Anderson, L. (1984c). Behavioral efficacy of haloperidol and lithium carbonate: A comparison in hospitalized aggressive children with conduct disorder. *Archives of General Psychiatry, 120,* 650–656.

Carlson, G. A., & Cantwell, D. P. (1980). Unmasking masked depression in children and adolescents. *American Journal of Psychiatry, 137,* 445–449.

Cohen, I. L., Campbell, M., Posner, D., Small, A. M., Triebel, D., & Anderson, L. T. (1980). Behavioral affects of haloperidol in young autistic children: An objective analysis using a within subjects reversal design. *Journal of the American Academy of Child Psychiatry, 19,* 665–677.

Conners, C. K. (1976). Classification and treatment of childhood depression and depressive equivalents. In D. Gallant & G. Simpson (Eds.), *Depression: Behavioral, biochemical, diagnostic, and treatment concepts* (pp. 181–204). New York: Spectrum.

Conners, C. K., Eisenberg, L., & Sharpe, L. (1964). Effect of methylphenidate in emotionally disturbed children. *Journal of Consulting Psychology, 28,* 14–22.

Cullinan, D., Epstein, M. H., & Kauffman, J. M. (1984). Teachers' ratings of students' behaviors: What constitutes behavior disorder in school? *Behavioral Disorders, 10,* 9–19.

DiMascio, A., Soltys, J. J., & Shader, R. I. (1970). *Psychotropic drug side effects.* Baltimore: Williams & Wilkins.

Eggers, G. (1978). Course and prognosis of childhood schizophrenia. *Journal of Autism and Childhood Schizophrenia, 1,* 21–35.

Engelhardt, D. M., Polizos, P., & Waizer, J. (1975). CNS consequences of psychotropic drug withdrawal in autistic children: A follow-up report. *Psychopharmacology Bulletin, 11,* 6–11.

Epstein, M. H., Cullinan, D., & Gadow, K. D. (1985). *Prevalence of psychotropic drug use with learning disabled, emotionally disturbed, and mentally retarded children.* Unpublished manuscript, Northern Illinois

University, Department of Learning, Development, and Special Education, DeKalb.

Fish, B. (1971). The "one child, one drug" myth of stimulants in hyperkinesis. *Archives of General Psychiatry, 25,* 193–203.

Fish, B. (1976). Pharmacotherapy for autistic and schizophrenic children. In E. R. Ritvo, B. J. Freeman, E. M. Ornitz, & P. E. Tanguay (Eds.), *Autism: Diagnosis, current research and treatment* (pp. 107–119). New York: Spectrum.

Fish, B., Campbell, M., Shapiro, T., & Floyd, A., Jr. (1969). Comparison of trifluperidol, trifluoperazine and chlorpromazine in preschool schizophrenic children: the value of less sedative antipsychotic agents. *Current Therapeutic Research, 11,* 589–595.

Fish, B., Shapiro, T., & Campbell, M. (1966). Long term prognosis and the response of schizophrenic children to drug therapy: A controlled study of trifluoperazine. *American Journal of Psychiatry, 123,* 32–39.

Freed, H., & Peifer, C. A. (1956). Treatment of hyperkinetic emotionally disturbed children with prolonged administration of chlorpromazine. *American Journal of Psychiatry, 13,* 22–26.

Freeman, L. N., Poznanski, E. O., Grossman, J. A., Buchsbaum, Y. Y., & Banegas, M. E. (1985). Psychotic and depressed children: A new entity. *Journal of the American Academy of Child Psychiatry, 24,* 95–102.

Geller, B., Chestnut, E. C., Miller, M. D., Price, D. T., & Yates, E. (1985). Preliminary data on DSM III associated features of major depressive disorder in children and adolescents. *American Journal of Psychiatry, 142,* 643–644.

Geller, B., Cooper, T. B., Chestnut, E., Abel, A. S., & Anker, J. A. (1984). Nortriptyline pharmacokinetic parameters in depressed children and adolescents: Preliminary data. *Journal of Clinical Psychopharmacology, 4,* 265–269.

Gillberg, C. (1984). Infantile autism and other childhood psychoses in a Swedish urban region. Epidemiologic aspects. *Journal of Child Psychology and Psychiatry, 25,* 35–43.

Gittelman-Klein, R., Klein, D. F., Katz, S., Saraf, K., & Pollack, E. (1976). Comparative effects of methylphenidate and thioridazine in hyperactive children. *Archives of General Psychiatry, 33,* 1217–1231.

Glazer, W., & Moore, D. C. (1981). A tardive dyskinesia clinic in a mental health center. *Hospital & Community Psychiatry, 32,* 572–574.

Graham, P. (1974). Depression in pre-pubertal children. *Developmental Medicine and Child Neurology, 16,* 340–349.

Green, W. H., Campbell, M., Hardesty, A. S., Grega, D. M., Padron-Gayol, M., Shell, J., & Erlenmeyer-Kimling, L. (1984). A comparison of schizophrenic and autistic children. *Journal of the American Academy of Child Psychiatry, 23,* 399–409.

Gualtieri, C. T., Quade, D., Hicks, R. E., Mayo, J. P., & Schroeder, S. R. (1984). Tardive dyskinesia and other clinical consequences of neuroleptic treatment in children and adolescents. *American Journal of Psychiatry, 141,* 20–23.

Guy, W. (Ed.). (1976). *ECDEU assessment manual for psychopharmacology.* Washington, DC: U.S. Government Printing Office.

Hartlage, L. C. (1965). Effects of chlorpromazine on learning. *Psychological Bulletin, 64,* 235–245.

Heuyer, G., Gerard, G., & Galibert, J. (1953). Traitement de l'excitation psychometrics chez l'enfant pare (le 4560 r.p.). *Archives Francaises de Pediatrie, 9*, 961.

Kalachnik, J. E. (1985). Applied aspects of tardive dyskinesia monitoring: Over, under, sideways down; backward, forward, square, and round. In K. D. Gadow (Ed.), *Advances in learning and behavioral disabilities* (Vol. 4, pp. 133–180). Greenwich, CT: JAI Press.

Kalachnik, J. E., Larum, J. G., & Swanson, A. (1983). A tardive dyskinesia monitoring policy for applied facilities. *Psychopharmacology Bulletin, 19*, 277–282.

Kalachnik, J. E., Young, R. C., & Offerman, D. (1984). A tardive dyskinesia evaluation and diagnosis form for applied facilities. *Psychopharmacology Bulletin, 20*, 303–308.

Kamm, I., & Mandel, A. (1967). Thioridazine in the treatment of behavior disorders in epileptics. *Diseases of the Nervous System, 28*, 46–48.

Kammerlohr, B., Henderson, R. A., & Rock, S. (1983). Special education due process hearings in Illinois. *Exceptional Children, 49*, 417–422.

Kashani, J. H., Shekim, W. O., & Reid, J. C. (1984). Amitriptyline in children with major depressive disorder: A double-blind crossover pilot study. *Journal of the American Academy of Child Psychiatry, 23*, 348–351.

Kashani, J., & Simonds, J. F. (1979). The incidence of depression in children. *American Journal of Psychiatry, 136*, 1203–1205.

Kashani, J. H., McGee, R. O., Clarkson, S. E., et al. (1983). Depression in a sample of 9-year-old children. *Archives of General Psychiatry, 40*, 1217–1223.

Katz, S., Saraf, K., Gittelman-Klein, R., & Klein, D. F. (1975). Clinical pharmacological management of hyperkinetic children. *International Journal of Mental Health, 4*, 157–181.

Klein, D. F., & Davis, J. M. (1969). *Diagnosis and drug treatment of psychiatric disorders.* Baltimore: Williams & Wilkins.

Klein, D. F., Gittelman, R., Quikin, F., & Rifkin, A. (1980). *Diagnosis and drug treatment of psychiatric disorders: Adults and children* (2nd ed.). Baltimore: Williams & Wilkins.

Kobayashi, R. (1977). Drug therapy of tardive dyskinesia. *New England Journal of Medicine, 296*, 257–260.

Kolvin, I., Berney, T. P., & Bhate, S. R. (1984). Classification and diagnosis of depression in school phobia. *British Journal of Psychiatry, 145*, 347–357.

Kovacs, M., Feinberg, T. L., Crouse-Novak, M. A., Paulauskas, S. L., & Finkelstein, R. (1984). Depressive disorders in childhood: I. A. longitudinal prospective study of characteristics and recovery. *Archives of General Psychiatry, 41*, 229–237.

Kydd, R. R., & Werry, J. S. (1982). Schizophrenia in children under 16 years. *Journal of Autism and Developmental Disorders, 12*, 343–357.

Loney, J., & Milich, R. (1982). Hyperactivity, inattention, and aggression in clinical practice. In M. Wolraich & D. K. Routh (Eds.), *Advances in behavioral pediatrics* (Vol. 2, pp. 113–147). Greenwich, CT: JAI Press.

McAndrew, J. B., Case, Q., & Treffert, D. A. (1972). Effects of prolonged phenothiazine intake on psychotic and other hospitalized children. *Journal of Autism and Childhood Schizophrenia, 2*, 75–91.

McCarthy, J. M., & Paraskevopoulos, J. (1969). Behavior patterns of learning disabled, emotionally disturbed, and average children. *Exceptional Children, 36,* 69–74.

Paulson, G. W., Rizvi, C. A., & Crane, G. E. (1975). Tardive dyskinesia as a possible sequel of long-term therapy with phenothiazines. *Clinical Pediatrics, 14,* 953–955.

Perry, R., Campbell, M., Grega, D. M., & Anderson, L. (1984). Saliva lithium level in children: Their use in monitoring serum lithium levels and lithium side effects. *Journal of Clinical Psychopharmacology, 4,* 199–202.

Petti, T. A., & Law, W. (1982). Imipramine treatment of depressed children: A double-blind pilot study. *Journal of Clinical Psychopharmacology, 2,* 107–110.

Physicians' Desk Reference (39th ed.). (1985). Oradell, NJ: Medical Economics.

Platt, J. E., Campbell, M., Green, W. H., & Grega, D. M. (1984). Cognitive effects of lithium carbonate and haloperidol in treatment-resistant aggressive children. *Archives of General Psychiatry, 120,* 657–662.

Polizos, P., Engelhardt, D. M., Hoffman, S. P., & Waizer, J. (1973). Neurological consequences of psychotic drug withdrawal in schizophrenic children. *Journal of Autism and Childhood Schizophrenia, 3,* 247–253.

Puig-Antich, J. (1982). Major depression and conduct disorder in prepuberty. *Journal of the American Academy of Child Psychiatry, 21,* 118–128.

Puig-Antich, J., Perel, J. M., Lupatkin, W., Chambers, W. J., Shea, C., Tabrizi, M. A., & Stiller, R. L. (1979). Plasma levels of imipramine (IMI) and desmethylimipramine (DMI) and clinical response in prepubertal major depressive disorder. *Journal of the American Academy of Child Psychiatry, 18,* 616–627.

Quay, H. C., Morse, W. C., & Cutler, R. L. (1966). Personality patterns of pupils in special classes for the emotionally disturbed. *Exceptional Children, 32,* 297–301.

Raiser, L., & Van Nagel, C. (1980). The loophole in Public Law 94–142. *Exceptional Children, 46,* 516–520.

Rapoport, J. (1976). Pediatric psychopharmacology and childhood depression. In D. F. Klein & R. Gittelman-Klein (Eds.), *Progress in psychiatric drug treatment* (Vol. 2, pp. 493–504). New York: Brunner/Mazel.

Rimland, B., Callaway, E., & Dreyfus, P. (1978). The effects of high doses of vitamin B_6 on autistic children: A double-blind crossover study. *American Journal of Psychiatry, 135,* 472–475.

Ritvo, E. R., Freeman, B. J., Geller, E., & Yuwiler, A. (1983). Effects of fenfluramine on 14 autistic outpatients. *Journal of the American Academy of Child Psychiatry, 22,* 549–558.

Rivera-Calimlim, L., Nasrallah, H., Strauss, J., & Lasagna, L. (1976). Clinical response and plasma levels: Effective dose, dosage schedules, and drug interactions on plasma chlorpromazine levels. *American Journal of Psychiatry, 133,* 646–652.

Rutter, M. (1972). Childhood schizophrenia reconsidered. *Journal of Autism and Childhood Schizophrenia, 2,* 315–337.

Rutter, M. (1985). The treatment of autistic children. *Journal of Child Psychology and Psychiatry, 26,* 193–214.

Rutter, M., Tizard, J., & Whitmore, K. (Eds.). (1970). *Education, health, and behavior.* London: Longmans.

Safer, D. J., & Krager, J. M. (1984). Trends in medication treatment of hyperactive school children. In K. D. Gadow (Ed.), *Advances in learning and behavioral disabilities* (Vol. 3, pp. 125–149). Greenwich, CT: JAI Press.

Schroeder, S. R., & Gualtieri, C. T. (1985). Behavioral interactions induced by chronic neuroleptic therapy in persons with mental retardation. *Psychopharmacology Bulletin, 21,* 310–315.

Sprague, R. L., Barnes, K. R., & Werry, J. S. (1970). Methylphenidate and thioridazine: Learning, reaction time, activity, and classroom behavior in emotionally disturbed children. *American Journal of Orthopsychiatry, 40,* 615–628.

Sprague, R. L., Kalachnik, J. E., Breuning, S. E., Davis, V. J., Ullman, R. K., Cullari, S., Davidson, N. A., Ferguson, D. G., Anderson, B., & Hoffer, B. S. (1984a). The Dyskinesia Identification System-Coldwater (DISCo): A tardive dyskinesia rating scale for the developmentally disabled. *Psychopharmacology Bulletin, 20,* 328–338.

Sprague, R. L., Kalachnik, J. E., & White, D. M. (1985). *Dyskinesia Identification System: Condensed User Scale (DISCUS).* University of Illinois, Institute for Child Behavior and Development, 51 Gerty Drive, Champaign, IL 61820.

Sprague, R. L., & Werry, J. S. (1974). Psychotropic drugs and handicapped children. In L. Mann & D. A. Sabatino (Eds.), *The second review of special education* (pp. 1–50). Philadelphia: JSE Press.

Sprague, R. L., White, D. M., Ullmann, R., & Kalachnik, J. E. (1984b). Methods for selecting items in a tardive dyskinesia rating scale. *Psychopharmacology Bulletin, 20,* 339–345.

Stewart, M. A., DeBlois, C. S., Meardon, J., & Cummings, C. (1980). Aggressive conduct disorder of children: The clinical picture. *Journal of Mental Disease, 168,* 604–610.

Werry, J. S., & Aman, M. G. (1975). Methylphenidate and haloperidol in children. *Archives of General Psychiatry, 32,* 790–795.

Whall, A. L., Engle, V., Edwards, A., Bobel, L., & Haberland, C. (1983). Development of a screening program for tardive dyskinesia: Feasibility issues. *Nursing Research, 32,* 151–156.

Williams, D. T., Mehl, R., Yudofsky, S., Adams, D., & Roseman, B. (1982). The effect of propranolol on uncontrolled rage outbursts in children and adolescents with organic brain dysfunction. *Journal of the American Academy Child Psychiatry, 21,* 129–135.

Winsberg, B. G., & Yepes, L. E. (1978). Antipsychotics. In J. S. Werry (Ed.), *Pediatric psychopharmacology: The use of behavior modifying drugs in children* (pp. 234–273). New York: Brunner/Mazel.

Winsberg, B. G., Yepes, L. E., & Bialer, I. (1976). Pharmacologic management of children with hyperactive/aggressive/inattentive behavior disorders. *Clinical Pediatrics, 15,* 471–477.

Wysocki, T., Fuqua, W., Davis, V. J., & Breuning, S. E. (1981). Effects of thioridazine (Mellaril) on titrating delayed matching-to-sample performance of mentally retarded adults. *American Journal of Mental Deficiency, 85,* 539–547.

Chapter **5**

Adolescent Psychiatric Disorders

John Pomeroy * *and*
Kenneth D. Gadow

The inclusion of a chapter solely on the treatment of adolescents with psychotropic medication is, surprisingly, an unusual phenomenon. Although professionals and lay persons have no difficulty in defining this stage of development as unique, there seems to be some reluctance (at least until quite recently) to separate younger adolescents from prepubertal children, and older adolescents from adults, when considering medical management. This chapter is intended to clarify the appropriateness of considering adolescents separately, present a rational approach to psychiatric diagnosis and treatment, and dispel some of the myths that abound in this area. Most of the topics discussed here are by necessity reviewed only briefly, but it is hoped that the interested reader will use the references cited to expand their knowledge. Two good sources of information are Berg's *Reading About Adolescence* (1984) and Rutter's *Changing Youths in a Changing Society* (1980). Although these clinicians are English, they provide an excellent source of scientific literature from both sides of the Atlantic Ocean.

ADOLESCENT DEVELOPMENT

Adolescence, as a phase of maturing from childhood to adulthood, has been recognized from classical times, but it is a relatively recent

---

*Dr. John Pomeroy, M.B.B.S. (London), M.R.C. Psych., Chief of Child Psychiatry Service, Health Sciences Center, State University of New York at Stony Brook.

notion that it differs in any marked way from the preceding or following years. In fact, modern concepts of childhood probably did
not originate until the 17th and 18th centuries (Anthony, 1982), and
cultural changes, such as increasing societal complexity, child labor
laws, and improved higher education, appear more influential in
defining this stage of development than the physical realities of maturation. Erikson (1968) has suggested that with these cultural
changes has come a need for a psychosocial "moratorium" to prepare the adolescent for the adult roles of the 20th century. It has
been argued that the prolonging of higher education for much larger
numbers of youths (particularly in the United States) is an important
factor in the increase in extent and force of the youth movement in
the last 30 years (Braungart, 1975).

G. Stanley Hall (1904) is generally considered to be the first
psychologist to conceptualize this developmental stage, and he
associated it with a time of strife and stress suggesting inherent
instability, emotional turmoil, and psychic disturbance. Enthusias-
tically endorsed by psychoanalytic theorists (Blos, 1970; Freud,
1958), psychiatric disturbance in adolescence came to be seen as
virtually normal. Diagnostic practice in the 1960s for adolescents
seen in American clinics reflected this assumption, and most disorders were considered transient adjustment problems (Rosen et al.,
1965).

In the last 20 years, empirical study has challenged many of
these initial impressions of adolescence. A more rational approach
to the interaction of biological, psychological, emotional, and social
changes has not only produced a more optimistic viewpoint of adolescence but initiated an understanding of the true problems that
occur.

Biological, Psychological, and Social Changes

Numerous physiological and biochemical processes are associated
with the attainment of physical maturity. The most overt changes are
a growth spurt and sexual maturation, which are set in motion by
hormonal changes that start between 18 and 24 months before the
first physical evidence of puberty. The peak age of increase in height
and weight is 11 to 12 years for girls and 14 years for boys. The
secondary sexual characteristics show the same pattern of earlier
development for girls.

Emotional reactions to these changes can be produced by many
mechanisms, including (a) the psychological need to adjust to radi-
cal development in shape and size and the assumption of functional
sexual ability, (b) the possible direct influence of hormonal changes,

and (c) comparison among peers of rates of development and appearance. Early maturing boys seem to be at some advantage intellectually and in personality (Graham & Rutter, 1973), but for girls the picture is less consistent.

There are also internal changes taking place that are of importance in our consideration of appropriate drug management. Associated with the growth spurt is a rapid increase in size and weight of the heart, an accelerated growth of the lungs, and a sudden decline in basal metabolism. In accompaniment with this there is a change in the relative proportions of water, fat, and other substances inside or outside the cells in the body. Subsequently, adolescents are likely to require *less* in weight-related doses of most drugs than younger children.

There are two major areas of psychological development in adolescence. One is in the thinking (cognitive) capacities and the other in emotional demands. Intellectual growth is obviously not going to be apparent in major changes in IQ scores, because this is a relative measure between individuals of the same age group. Cognitive skills, however, show rapid change in reasoning, creativity, and learning abilities.

Numerous theories and descriptions of the development of thinking capacity have evolved. It appears that development occurs more rapidly for biological capabilities (related to nervous system maturation), such as perceptual speed, than those associated with experience, such as word fluency. The most influential writer in the area of cognitive development, Piaget, describes the crucial intellectual change as the growth of logical reasoning or "formal operations" (Inhelder & Piaget, 1958). This makes it possible for the adolescent to understand different perspectives, use abstract concepts, and develop testable hypotheses. Such changes are seen in the "testing out" of ideas and beliefs that are typical of the adolescent.

Because adolescence is a time to gradually relinquish the security and dependence of childhood and to develop independence and personal identity, this produces another set of psychological changes. This process, with its pain and stress, can often lead to unpredictable and apparently inexplicable behavior. The so-called rebellion of youth can be seen as a necessary rejection of adult values, making it easier to give them up. The sense of emptiness and loss that can follow this new found independence is probably another measure of the ambivalence of the adolescent experience. How these emotional changes relate to psychiatric disturbance is discussed later.

In association with biological and psychological disruption, the developing adolescent is subjected to numerous social pressures from adults and peers. Parental expectations may include improved educational performance and less dependence, but at the same time, the adolescent must adopt new roles in the transition from child to adult. These may well occur before the adolescent feels ready or be delayed against his or her wishes. The latter results in the conflict between adult standards and peer expectation, which is typically manifested in disagreements over topics such as curfew and dress.

Adolescent Turmoil

As previously stated, much has been written about the changes and potential problems that occur for the normal adolescent, which has led to the expectation that adolescents must go through a period of turbulence for normal growth. However, studies of large numbers of adolescents (e.g., Offer & Offer, 1975; Rutter et al., 1976) have corrected many of these preconceptions. The weight of evidence now points to the fact that the majority of adolescents do *not* experience an identity crisis, become shy and withdrawn, or become alienated from their parents. It is true to say that about half the adolescent population experiences sadness, anxiety, and self-consciousness, but the majority find appropriate coping mechanisms to deal with these feelings.

As a generalization it can be stated that those characteristics once said to be a part of normal adolescence (withdrawal, conduct problems, antisocial behavior, prolonged depression) are more likely to be indicators of psychosocial or psychiatric disturbance. This reality is highlighted by findings that disturbed adolescents do not seem to outgrow their problems (Masterson, 1967). Moreover, of those diagnosed as having *situational disorder* (temporary psychological disturbance caused by external stressors), at least half continue to require psychiatric care at the same rate as those given formal psychiatric diagnoses (Weiner & Del Gaudio, 1976) or prove to have more serious psychiatric disturbances (Andreason & Hoenk, 1982).

Before dismissing all the common beliefs about adolescence, it is worth pointing out that there have been significant social changes in recent decades. For example, in the 1970s youths were more politically liberal, more active sexually, less oriented toward organized religion, and less success-oriented than previous generations of adolescents (Bengston & Starr, 1975). The importance of this "gap" is unclear because differences in attitude can be found between adolescents who are only 1 year apart in age (Baltes & Nesselroade, 1972). Social problems for adolescents such as sexually transmitted diseases, abortion, illegitimate births, drug abuse, alcoholism, delinquency, vandalism, suicide, and attempted suicide have all shown a rapid increase in the last 30 years up to the end of the 1970s (Rutter, 1980).

It seems apparent that the present day is a difficult time for many adolescents, but it is helpful to keep an historical perspective. For example, the suicide rate in late 19th century Saxony for children and adolescents was 10 times the rate for the United States in the 1950s. Moreover, two out of five suicides in Moscow during the years 1908 and 1909 were of children or adolescents (Bakwin, 1957).

PSYCHIATRIC SYNDROMES IN ADOLESCENCE

Because psychological problems of adolescence do not necessarily represent natural maturational processes, it is necessary to know how true psychiatric disorders are defined. Adult psychiatrists are most likely to use a diagnostic approach known as syndromal. This implies that patients can be classified by a number of symptoms that tend to go commonly together to produce a definition of a disorder. The formulation of syndromes is useful because it enables clinicians to communicate effectively about the symptoms of illness. It also provides a structure for learning more about the course, treatment, outcome, and cause of the disorder. Ideal as this is for general medical conditions such as infectious diseases, it has not always been a comfortable approach for psychiatric disturbance. However, terms such as schizophrenia, major depression, and obsessive-compulsive disorder do tend to fulfill many of the requirements of a syndrome.

In child psychiatry dealing with prepubertal children, diagnosis is more related to a cluster of behavioral observations (e.g., overactivity, aggression, withdrawal) by parents, teachers, and clinicians. The type of behavior and the degree to which it exceeds normal standards for similar-aged peers determines the diagnostic group in which the child's disturbance is placed. There is some variation in diagnostic practices for children from one country to the next, and many epidemiological studies merely define children's disorders as conduct, emotional, or mixed. The system formulated by the American Psychiatric Association (1980) is more inclined to break these larger groupings into smaller groups that appear similar to the syndromes of adult psychiatry, for example, attention deficit disorder, separation anxiety, and withdrawal disorder. Each of these disorders is associated with a set of criteria for making a diagnosis, but there is much controversy surrounding this and all other diagnostic systems.

Adolescent psychiatric disorders can also be differentiated with regard to when the youth's problems first become serious enough to require special help. Some adolescents, for example, are likely to experience problems because their childhood behavioral difficulties continue into adolescence (e.g., hyperactivity). Others develop major problems for the first time during adolescence, some of which may resemble childhood disorders (e.g., conduct disorder), whereas others resemble adult psychiatric syndromes. These observations raise a number of questions.

1. What Happens to Childhood Disorders in Adolescence?

There is strong evidence that a large number of adolescent psychiatric disorders have their origins in childhood. This is more apparent in adolescents who are treated in psychological clinics than it is in troubled adolescents who are identified in surveys of the general population (Capes et al., 1971; Rutter et al., 1976). Continuity for disturbance is stronger for conduct disorders than emotional disorders (except psychosis), but all disorders that continue from childhood into adolescence tend to remain clinically similar through the years. Things that are associated with continuing pathology from childhood are family disruptions and learning problems. Adolescent psychiatric disorders that begin in childhood are more likely to be present in boys (about 2:1), whereas disorders that begin for the first time in adolescence are equally common in males and females, although specific disorders may be associated more with one sex than another.

Not only do many psychiatric disorders originate in childhood and continue into adolescence, but clinical changes can occur. For example, approximately 20% of all autistic children develop seizure disorders in adolescence. Among the disorders that may show clinical change over time are the three major groups discussed in this book: hyperactivity, seizure disorders, and mental retardation. The more severe cases in childhood often present somewhat greater problems in adolescence. Part of this may be a reaction to their inherent handicaps, or they become more of a management problem owing to their increased size and independence. Some disorders decrease significantly in prevalence in adolescence, such as enuresis and encopresis, but when they do continue, they may signify more severe pathology.

2. What Disorders First Occur in Adolescence?

Of the psychiatric disorders that first begin in adolescence, many show a steady rise in prevalence through the adolescent period, but fortunately they remain fairly rare. These include the behavioral problems of school refusal, suicide, and severe aggression and the psychiatric syndromes of schizophrenia, obsessive-compulsive disorders, and phobic states. More common are depressive states, attempted suicide, alcoholism, drug abuse, and eating disorders.

3. Are Adolescent Disorders Related to Age?

The psychiatric problems of adolescents show changes in character and prevalence dependent on age, and it is convenient to think of three stages:

A. Early adolescence (11 to 14 years): Minor problems center on issues of impulse control. School refusal and depression increase in frequency, and for boys particularly, conduct problems such as lying, stealing, and truanting predominate. Epidemiological studies suggest that 14-year-olds have psychiatric problems at two to three times the 10-year-old rate.
B. Midadolescence (14 to 17 years): Minor problems commonly relate to concerns about identity. Adult-type syndromal disorders begin to emerge (e.g., schizophrenia, mood disorders), but they are more variable. In girls attempted suicide, pregnancy, and eating disorders predominate, whereas in boys conduct problems, drug abuse, and academic failure are more noticeable. Sexual problems such as fears of the consequences of masturbation, homosexual concerns, and occasionally more perverse sexual acting out can occur.
C. Late adolescence (17 to 21 years): Problems relate to establishing oneself vocationally and socially. Mood disturbance, anxiety states, and phobic disorders are common, especially in girls. Psychiatric disorders increase in frequency, and there is some evidence of greater stress for those continuing into higher education.

Special Problems of Treating Adolescents

Adolescents' social and behavioral problems cause considerable anxiety for others, but teenagers do not always agree that they are in need of help. The initial problems are identifying individuals in need of assessment, helping them accept intervention, and using

appropriate diagnostic approaches to delineate the correct treatment. Errors can occur when the therapist either becomes too
strongly identified with parental or societal authorities and subsequently alienates the adolescent or tends to accept the adolescent's
behavior as purely a developmental norm when it is really a manifestation of pathology. Understanding the latter requires an ability to
separate the psychological problems of the adolescent from the
social, family, and other environmental factors that might produce
or exacerbate symptoms and hence lead to a referral to a psychological or psychiatric clinic.

Just because an adolescent is having serious problems does not
necessarily mean that medication is appropriate, especially if it prevents the youth and the family from taking responsibility for behavior within their control. In those cases where medication is
warranted, it is rarely a cure (such as penicillin is for streptococcal
infections). Medication is often used to help with particular target
symptoms (e.g., aggression, impulse control, anxiety) or as an aid
during crisis before other interventions such as psychotherapy can
be instituted. When medication is used, the trusting relationship
between the psychiatrist and adolescent is crucial, because noncompliance (not taking medication as directed) can be a major problem.

The use of medication for psychiatric problems in children and
adolescents remains controversial, and research suggests that it is
slightly more common in American than European child psychiatric
practice. There are many attempts to evaluate the benefits of medication scientifically, but the reader should realize that medications are
only one aspect of the treatment approaches used in child and adolescent psychiatry. Other treatments include cognitive, behavioral,
and insight-oriented therapies with individuals, groups, and families as well as environmental manipulations such as change of
school placement, residential treatment, and social interventions.

Specific Uses of Psychotropic Medicine

Because medication is often used in adolescent psychiatric practice
to help with target symptoms that reflect abnormal functioning,
treatment is discussed for disorders involving the following areas of
functioning: mood (depression, mania), thinking (psychosis), conduct (aggression, hyperactivity), eating (anorexia nervosa, bulimia,
obesity), and emotions (anxiety, phobias, obsessional disorders).
More emphasis is placed on the drugs that are not described in other
sections of this book or where specific information about studies
with adolescents is available.

DISORDERS OF MOOD

As stated earlier, *transient* (short-lived) mood changes of little long-term significance are common in adolescents. However, there is also a significant rise in the rate of mood-related psychiatric illnesses during this period. These disorders are characterized by a significant and persistent alteration in mood, which is accompanied by biological and behavioral changes. Biological symptoms such as sleep and eating disturbances mainly define the illness and differentiate it from a reactive or temporary change in mood.

Table 5–1 shows the major characteristics that are considered in a childhood and adolescent diagnosis of an abnormally elevated mood (*mania*) and an abnormally lowered mood (*depression*). These diagnostic criteria were originally formulated by Weinberg and Brumback (1976) for prepubertal children and later modified by Hassanyeh and Davison (1980) for a study of adolescents. The American Psychiatric Association's (1980) diagnostic criteria for *major depressive disorder* appear in Table 4–5 (Emotional Disturbance). Although mania is considerably less common, it can occur in adolescents and is part of a special type of mood disorder known as *bipolar affective disorder* (or *manic-depressive illness*). In such cases, phases or cycles of illness are seen in which either mania or depression are manifested. The most common mood disorder is *unipolar depressive illness*, that is, the youth only experiences depression. Both bipolar and unipolar disorders have characteristics that suggest that the individual is genetically or, in some way, physiologically predisposed. Adolescents who experience these problems suffer recurring, intermittent disturbances that may or may not be related to external precipitants (e.g., death in the family, poor school grades), but the disorder itself is believed to have an organic basis.

Diagnosis is complicated by the fact that the symptoms of mood disorders vary so greatly in teenagers and includes such items as refusal to go to school, social withdrawal, deteriorating academic performance, unexplained conduct disturbance, and antisocial behaviors. Severe depression can result in *stupor* (a mute, withdrawn state often confused with neurologic disorders) or suicide attempts. Manic adolescents often appear overactive and overtalkative and can embroil themselves in unusual antisocial acts (e.g., driving the family car without a license) that lead to a diagnosis of conduct disorder. The alternative picture is one of *acute psychosis*, which is characterized by the above behavioral changes in combination with hallucinations, delusions, or unusual ideation. This latter group of symptoms may be mistakenly diagnosed as schizophrenia.

Table 5–1.   Clinical Criteria Employed by Hassanyeh and Davidson (1980) for Diagnosis of Mania and Depression in Adolescents

Mania = either or both 1 and 2 plus 3 or more from 3 to 8	*Depression* = both 1 and 2 plus 2 or more from 3 to 12
1. Euphoria	1. Depressed mood
2. Irritability	2. Self-depreciation (thoughts are negative and place emphasis on individual's faults)
3. Hyperactivity	
4. Pressure of speech (excessive, rapid speech)	3. Agitation (restless and extremely anxious)
5. Flight of ideas (rapid switching of ideas with some association between them)	4. Sleep disturbance
	5. Diminished school performance
	6. Diminished socialization
6. Grandiosity (false beliefs in having important powers or being an important person)	7. Change in attitude toward school
	8. Somatic complaints (complaints of physical symptoms)
7. Sleep disturbance	9. Loss of usual energy
8. Distractibility	10. Loss of appetite and/or weight
	11. Suicidal ideation (thoughts of killing or harming self)
	12. Psychomotor retardation (slowing down of thinking and movement)

It is important to realize that the depressive (and occasionally manic) symptoms are often observed in association with environmental stress (e.g., death of a loved one), drug and alcohol abuse, physical illness, and other psychiatric disorders. Focusing treatment on the depressive symptoms instead of the youth's problems may be ineffective or even detrimental.

Medical treatment for serious mood disorders is recommended for all age groups. Although these disorders are self-limiting, appropriate medical management significantly reduces the length and severity of disturbance and the risk of harm either through self-neglect or suicide. Management consists of both therapy for the acute illness and long-term treatment for prevention of recurrence.

Drug Therapy

Antidepressant medication consists largely of two major groups of drugs: the tricyclics and MAOIs (monoamine oxidase inhibitors). Newer antidepressants have been developed, but none seem likely to replace the drugs in either of these two categories as the primary agent for the management of mood disorders at this time.

The best indicators that a depressed adolescent will respond to antidepressant medication are the so-called vegetative (biological) symptoms such as sleep disturbance and lack of drive, particularly if there is also a family history of depression. Most studies of antidepressants for childhood depression have focused on the prepubertal child. Of the few reports pertaining entirely to adolescents, most generally recommended treating them the same way one would manage depressed adults (e.g., Esman, 1981).

Tricyclics. The commonest treatment is with tricyclic medication, particularly Tofranil (imipramine). Elavil (amitriptyline) is the second most commonly used tricyclic drug, although the package insert states that its use with children under 12 years old is not recommended (generally because there is insufficient research). In adolescents the appropriate dosage of Tofranil for depression ranges from 75 to 200 mg per day (often administered as a single dose at night), and it is possible to measure the level of drug in the blood, if required, to ensure a therapeutic level. Because there is a delay in the onset of an antidepressant effect, it will take at least 4 weeks before the response to medication can be adequately evaluated.

Tricyclic antidepressants often produce unwanted side effects that are troubleshome but rarely dangerous. These include dry mouth, drowsiness, nausea, blurred vision, constipation, and very rarely an inability to pass urine (*urinary retention*). Another major complication is its effect on nerve conduction within the heart muscle. Therapeutic levels of the tricyclics can produce changes in heart function that register on EKG records, and susceptible individuals may develop unusual heart rhythms or a "racing" of the heart (*tachycardia*). During treatment it is therefore imperative for the physician to assess heart function thoroughly. This effect on the heart is one of the main reasons why these drugs can be very lethal in overdose (accidental or not), which is an important consideration when using these drugs with children, particularly those with suicidal ideas. A more rare side effect of the tricyclics is the development of epileptic seizures, which appear to be associated with higher doses of medication.

The effects of tricyclic medication on cognitive and academic performance have not been studied extensively, but most reports with children are encouraging. The tricyclics have some actions that are similar to the stimulants, which probably account for the beneficial effects in some hyperactive children. These drugs can increase attention span and decrease impulsivity (Rapoport et al., 1974; Yepes et al., 1977). There is also evidence that long-term tricyclic treatment does not cause deterioration in academic performance (Quinn & Rapoport, 1975).

When adolescents respond to tricyclic antidepressants, there is a need to consider how long treatment should be continued. Mood disorders have a risk of recurrence, and evidence in adult studies suggests that treatment should be maintained for 3 to 6 months after full recovery. This policy also seems practical for adolescents. Reduction of the medication should be gradual because there is a potential for withdrawal symptoms (sleep disturbance, nightmares, and physical complaints) to occur if medication is stopped abruptly. Occasionally, adolescents with bipolar disorders "switch" to mania during the course of treatment with an antidepressant. This is an indication to withdraw the antidepressant medication and use an antimanic drug. At the present time there is some controversy as to whether the "switch" occurs owing to the antidepressant drug or whether it is purely a part of the illness process.

MAOIs. There are several MAOIs available for medical use of which Nardil (phenelzine) is the most commonly used. They are considered to act as antidepressants because they inhibit an enzyme that breaks down certain chemical transmitters within the nervous system. The MAOIs are more commonly used in adults as the drug of second choice for depression because (a) they are associated with more troublesome side effects, and (b) early reports indicate that they were more effective in anxiety-related disorders (e.g., phobic states, obsessive-compulsive disorders), particularly if there are also mild symptoms of depression. More recent reports suggest that inadequate dosages have accounted for the belief that they are not effective antidepressants and that the risks of treatment are possibly exaggerated. Even so, it remains true to say that in adolescents there are few, if any, indications for their use except in intractable (difficult to control) depressions and severe emotional disorders (which are described later in the chapter).

The medical literature on the use of MAOIs with adolescents consists of anecdotal reports or poorly controlled studies. The side effects of these drugs are usually few, but include nausea, dizziness, and sleep disturbance, particularly if given later in the day. The main concern is the potential for life-threatening reactions when treated individuals eat food containing tyramine (e.g., matured cheeses, yeast products) or are given a number of different medications. The combination of MAOIs and these substances can produce a rapid rise in blood pressure because the normal biochemical mechanism for breaking down these chemicals has been inhibited by the drug. It is therefore important that the adolescent who is administered an MAOI (a) takes medication in the prescribed manner, (b) follows all dietary restrictions, and (c) avoids illicit drugs, particularly, cocaine and amphetamine (speed).

Lithium. Antimanic agents that are most commonly used are of two major types, the neuroleptics and lithium salts (usually lithium carbonate). Both groups of drugs are effective in the acute stage of mania, although the neuroleptics generally have a more rapid calming effect. Lithium is also effective in reducing the recurrence of mood disorder in individuals prone to bipolar affective disorder. More recently, there has been an interest in a wider application of lithium in adolescent patients (see also the section on Conduct Disorder). Because the therapeutic effect of the neuroleptics is presumably the same as in any acute psychosis, they are discussed in the next section.

The increasing use of lithium in adolescent psychiatry is attested to by a number of recent review articles on this topic (Campbell et al., 1978; Steinberg, 1980; Youngerman & Canino, 1978). Although noted in the 1940s to be a possible treatment for manic excitement, it was not until the 1960s in Scandinavia that the beneficial effects of lithium were really tested. One of the difficulties of using the drug is that there is a narrow range between therapeutic drug levels and toxic levels. This means that regular measurements of the level of lithium in the blood are necessary.

Lithium is effective in treating mania, but in the initial phase of illness, it is commonly given in combination with a neuroleptic because the neuroleptic will help the adolescent calm down. Haldol (haloperidol) is *not* recommended to be used in combination with lithium because there are a few reports of brain damage in patients taking both these drugs. Long-term treatment with lithium is considered appropriate when (a) there is clear evidence of recurring episodes of mood disorder and they are occurring often and (b) they are disruptive enough to warrant the risks of long-term treatment. Dosage is generally in the range of 1,000 to 1,600 mg per day, but the true measure of dosage is the amount of lithium necessary to keep the level in the blood within the known therapeutic range. Adolescents reportedly tolerate larger doses of lithium because they tend to excrete lithium through their kidneys more rapidly than older adults.

The side effects of lithium include nausea, fine *tremor* (slight trembling or shaking, usually of the hands), thirst, excessive need to urinate *(polyuria)*, and loose stools. Signs of toxicity are vomiting, diarrhea, shaking, sleepiness, slurred speech, and dizziness. Concerns about long-term adverse reactions include potentially irreversible effects on the kidney, thyroid, and possibly bone. None of these problems have proved to be common and can be easily monitored by regular testing of chemical and hormonal levels in the blood.

The effects of lithium on cognitive function are unclear. In normal volunteers, lithium can induce apathy, impair word learning, and reduce performance on visual-motor tasks, but studies of patients on long-term lithium therapy have found no impairment on standardized intelligence test performance. It seems reasonable to conclude that for adolescents with severe recurrent mood disorder, neither side effects nor fear of cognitive deterioration are sufficient reasons not to use lithium in appropriate cases.

Tegretol (Carbamazepine). This antiepileptic drug (see Chapter 2) has become of considerable interest to psychiatrists in the last decade. Initial reports of an antimanic effect of Tegretol (Ballenger & Post, 1978) have been followed by more rigorous studies that confirm that the drug is useful in the treatment of mania and *rapid-cycling mood disorders* (prolonged mood disturbance with rapid switches between mania and depression) and for long-term treatment to prevent mood disorder (Kishimoto et al., 1983; Roy-Byrne et al., 1984a). In the study by Kishimoto there was evidence that Tegretol was more effective in patients with an onset of bipolar affective disorder before the age of 20 years.

At the present time Tegretol is used largely for lithium-resistant patients. Therapeutic dosages are similar to those for the treatment of seizure disorders and are usually based on measurement of drug level in the blood. Combination therapy of lithium and Tegretol has been reported as beneficial, but there remains uncertainty whether this combination can produce a toxic reaction in the nervous system (Shukla et al., 1984).

Electroconvulsive Therapy

The induction of epileptic seizures by electric stimulation of the brain has been a controversial procedure since its introduction in the 1930s. However, modern procedure with anesthesia, muscle relaxation, and controlled application of current has produced a safe and effective treatment for severe, intractable mood disturbance. Isolated reports of its use in adolescent depression (Warneke, 1975) and mania (Carr et al., 1983) exist, and it seems likely that it will remain in the armamentarium of treatment for adolescents when the mood disorder is extreme and unresponsive to known drug therapy or when medication is contraindicated because of side effects or complicating health problems.

DISORDERS OF THINKING

Disorders of thinking are characterized by unusual and alien sensory perceptions (*hallucinations,* e.g., hearing voices that are not real), misinterpretation of the environment (*delusions,* e.g., the belief that people are following or conspiring against them), or jumbled and disjointed thinking (*thought disorder,* e.g., rambling or pointless speech, failure to keep a train of thought). Individuals with such symptoms, often in combination with many other behavioral changes (e.g., sleep problems, overactivity or underactivity, social withdrawal or very inappropriate social behavior) are said to be suffering from *psychosis.*

In early childhood the term psychosis has also been attached to severe disturbances in development such as *infantile autism* (see Chapter 4). These disorders are probably not related to the psychoses seen in adolescence and do not respond in any dramatic way to neuroleptic medication. In early and middle childhood, neuroleptics are used primarily for behavioral management of severe conduct problems, whatever the underlying psychiatric diagnosis.

The psychotic states seen in adolescence are more likely to be due to (a) the effects of licit or illicit drugs or (b) represent a clinical manifestation of the *functional psychoses* (schizophrenia and bipolar affective psychosis). Although diagnosis is of importance, the management of the acute and often agitated psychotic state is the same, and the neuroleptics are used to calm the individual and reduce the psychotic phenomenon. The need for long-term drug treatment is based on diagnosis and is usually only recommended in the small number of adolescents diagnosed as having schizophrenia.

Schizophrenia is a life-long disorder with variable severity and degree of social, behavioral, and intellectual deterioration. *Florid* (active, easily observed) psychotic symptoms (e.g., hallucinations and delusions) occur in some stage of the illness and are not related to mood disturbance or gross abnormality of brain functioning (e.g., head injury, drug or alcohol abuse). The types of delusions and hallucinations vary, but those most associated with schizophrenia are listed in the diagnostic criteria devised by the American Psychiatric Association (1980) (Table 5–2). In addition to the florid symptoms, there is chronic evidence of personality change, usually expressed as an observable atypical mood (*abnormal affect*), which can show no modulation or range (*blunted, flat*) or be entirely inappropriate to the context of the situation (e.g., laughing about very sad events). Other characteristics are a social withdrawal, lack of

Table 5–2. DSM-III Diagnostic Criteria for Schizophrenic Disorder[a]

In accompaniment with a deterioration from a previous level of functioning and at least six months of continuous illness, at least one of the following should be present during a phase of the illness:

1. Bizarre delusions—content is patently absurd and has no possible basis in fact
2. Somatic, grandiose, religious, nihilistic or other delusions without persecutory or jealous content
3. Delusions with persecutory or jealous content if accompanied by hallucinations of any type
4. Auditory hallucinations in which either a voice keeps up a running commentary on the individual's behavior or thoughts or two or more voices converse with each other
5. Auditory hallucinations on several occasions with content of more than one or two words, having no apparent relation to depression or elation
6. Incoherence, marked loosening of association, markedly illogical thinking or marked poverty of content of speech with at least one of the following:

   a. blunted, flat, or inappropriate affect
   b. delusions or hallucinations
   c. catatonic or other grossly disorganized behavior

All of the above should have occurred without evidence of major mood disorder or organic mental disorder.

[a]American Psychiatric Association. (1980). *Diagnostic and statistical manual of mental disorders* (3rd ed.). Washington, DC: Author.

purpose, and failure to reach potential socially or vocationally. One particular type of schizophrenia, *catatonia*, is characterized by motor abnormalities as the most prominent symptoms. These may be a mute (does not talk), withdrawn state in which abnormal postures might be maintained for many hours or any extreme, excitable, uncontrolled, overactive state. When the motor problems have improved, the more classical schizophrenic thought abnormalities usually become more detectable.

Drug Therapy

Although there are five groups of neuroleptics (see Appendix A), there is rarely a need to use more than a few of the manufactured drugs in regular clinical practice. There are some medical reports about the use of neuroleptics with adolescents, particularly Thorazine (chlorpromazine), Mellaril (thioridazine), Stelazine (trifluoperazine), and Navane (thiothixene). For long-term treatment there is an oily suspension of a phenothiazine, Prolixin (fluphenazine decanoate), which can be administered intramuscularly with injections every 2 to 3 weeks. Because a full review of dosages, indications, and problems with the use of neuroleptics is presented in Chapter 4 (Emotional Disturbance), only a brief overview is presented here.

The effect of the various neuroleptic drugs is very similar, but the effective dosage varies considerably. Neuroleptics can be separated into a high dose—low potency group (e.g., Thorazine and Mellaril) and low dose—high potency group (e.g., Stelazine and Haldol). Although these categories are not important from the standpoint of antipsychotic effects, they are useful with regard to side effects (Table 5–3). In general, the high dose—low potency drugs are more often associated with sedation, a side effect of neuroleptic medication. This can sometimes be used to clinical advantage. For example, a highly agitated, restless patient will probably be better treated with Thorazine than Stelazine because the former is significantly more sedating. For adolescent schizophrenics in need of long-term treatment, the use of a low dose–high potency drug may be beneficial because it is less likely to reduce social and academic performance as a result of sedation (Realmuto et al., 1984).

In adolescence, the unwanted effects of these drugs have to be weighed against the severity of psychiatric disturbance. For example, a minor deterioration in intellectual performance is much less clinically relevant when confronted with a patient who is experiencing hallucinations and delusions and who will be institutionalized unless treated with neuroleptic medication. The management of acute (short-term) psychosis raises few concerns about the use of neuroleptics. Side effects such as sedation, dry mouth, blurred vision, dizziness, constipation, and the *acute extrapyramidal syndromes* (Parkinsonian syndrome, akathisia, and dystonia; see Chapter 4) are all self-limiting and reversible or, in the case of the acute extrapyramidal syndromes, treatable with anticholinergic drugs. The major clinical problem is for adolescents who require chronic or long-term treatment. Unfortunately, the findings from one study suggest that adolescent schizophrenics have a *poor* response to neuroleptics (Welner et al., 1979). Moreover, long-term neuroleptic treatment *may* cause a potentially irreversible movement disorder *(tardive dyskinesia)* in some patients as well as produce changes in hormone secretions and deterioration in cognitive performance.

Tardive dyskinesia usually occurs after many months of neuroleptic treatment and normally begins with uncontrolled rhythmic movements of lips and tongue, which may later proceed to affect the limbs and trunk. A similar reaction is often seen on stopping drug treatment, particularly in young patients. These abnormalities generally improve after the drug has been completely withdrawn but can continue indefinitely. Tardive dyskinesia does occur in adoles-

Table 5–3. Selected Neuroleptic Drugs: Adult Doses and Side Effects

Generic name	Trade name	Daily oral dose Usual (mg)	Daily oral dose Extreme* (mg)	Sedative effects	Extrapyramidal effects	Hypotensive effects
1. Phenothiazines						
Acetophenazine	Tindal	60–120	20–600	+ +	+ +	+
Chlorpromazine	Thorazine	300–800	25–2000	+ + +	+ +	+ +
Fluphenazine	Prolixin	2.5–20	1–30	+	+ + +	+
Mesoridazine	Serentil	75–300	24–400			
Perphenazine	Trilafon	8–32	4–64	+ +	+ +	+
Piperacetazine	Quide	20–160	5–200			
Prochlorperazine	Compazine	75–100	15–150	+ +	+ + +	+ +
Thioridazine	Mellaril	200–600	50–800	+ + +	+	+ +
Trifluoperazine	Stelazine	6–20	2–60	+	+ + +	+ +
Triflupromazine	Vesprin	100–150	50–300	+ +	+ + +	+ +
2. Thioxanthenes						
Chlorprothixene	Taractan	50–400	30–600	+ + +	+ +	+ +
Thiothixene	Navane	6–30	6–60	+ to + +	+ +	+ +
3. Others						
Haloperidol	Haldol	6–20	2–100	+	+ + +	+
Loxapine	Loxitane	60–100	20–250	+	+ +	+
Molidone	Moban	50–225	15–400	+ +	+	0

*Extreme dosage ranges are occasionally exceeded cautiously and only when appropriate measures have failed.

Note. From "Drugs and the Treatment of Psychiatric Disorders" by R. J. Baldessarini, in *The Pharmacological Basis of Therapeutics* (6th ed., pp. 408–411) by A. G. Gilman, L. S. Goodman, and A. Gilman (Eds.), 1980, New York: Macmillan. Copyright 1980 by Macmillan Publishing Co. Adapted by permission.

cents (Gualtieri et al., 1980) and should be an indicator for reviewing the need for medication. Gualtieri and co-workers (1984) showed that 18 children and adolescents in a group of 41 with mixed psychiatric diagnoses, all being treated with long-term neuroleptics, developed dyskinetic symptoms after their medication was stopped. More importantly, however, only 12 required a resumption of their neuroleptic treatment after a prolonged trial without medication. Unfortunately, no information about specific diagnoses is given, but the study raises concerns about the assumed need for long-term neuroleptic use.

Two recent studies have paid particular consideration to adolescent schizophrenics on long-term neuroleptic therapy. The first (Apter et al., 1983) examined the effects of Thorazine (treatment for at least 6 months) on male hormone production in 10 schizophrenic males who were between 15 to 18 years old. Not only was the male hormone (testosterone) level reduced in the blood, but the central brain mechanisms that control the release of the hormone were also suppressed. Other aspects of the study suggested that these reactions were reversible, but the effects on fertility and potency from longer treatment remain to be studied. Erickson et al. (1984) conducted the only study that specifically explored the effects of neuroleptic treatment on cognitive performance in adolescent schizophrenics. They found that neuroleptics did not improve attention (which is also true for adult schizophrenics) and that sedation was a serious problem for most of the subjects.

At the present time, the use of long-term neuroleptic treatment should be carefully considered. If the adolescent disorder is significantly improved with medication, it may only be a matter of trying to maintain the lowest dose and using the low dose–high potency drugs when possible. The development of serious side effects (e.g., tardive dyskinesia) usually necessitates a withdrawal of medication, and other approaches to treatment will have to be reviewed. In the case of schizophrenic disorders, social and vocational intervention are a crucial aspect of treatment, and reliance on medication solely is not likely to be effective.

DISORDERS OF CONDUCT: HYPERACTIVITY AND AGGRESSION

Conduct problems are a major cause of referral to child psychiatrists and include a large number of different characteristics (e.g., stealing, lying, running away, using illicit drugs, destroying property), which are often attributable to the adolescent's environment. Hyperactivity and aggression, however, are thought to be more biologically determined characteristics. For these reasons and the level of disruption these behaviors cause, drug therapy for adolescent conduct disorders has focused on aggression and the sequelae of childhood hyperactivity.

Aggression refers to a number of behaviors that are directed against another person, object, or self, and the main purpose is to establish some position of control or superiority. The feelings associated with the behavior are usually anger, hostility, rage, or fear. Developmentally, there is a reduction in the rate of aggression from early to middle childhood; also, aggression largely changes from undirected (temper) outbursts in the 2- to 4-year range to retaliatory and instrumental aggression in middle childhood (Goodenough, 1931). From a longitudinal perspective, there is evidence that from the age of 3 years, aggressivity as a trait is a very stable characteristic into adolescence (Farrington, 1978; Kagan & Moss, 1962; Manning et al., 1978). Although adolescent aggression is commonly a reaction to frustration, clinicians are often consulted when it is associated with neurologic conditions (e.g., mental retardation, seizure disorders, other organic brain disease such as the long-term effects of trauma, tumors, or infections), and particularly when the outbursts are reportedly out of the control of the individual. In such situations it is often true that behavioral interventions, teaching self-control, and psychosocial therapies fail to reduce the aggressive behavior.

Adolescent aggression may not only be related to neurodevelopmental abnormalities but also to character disturbance and other psychiatric disorders, such as depression, psychosis, or anxiety. There is also some overlap between adolescent aggression and childhood hyperactivity. The outcome of children with hyperactivity seems to be variable and is probably less optimistic than early reports, which suggested that children showed maturation leading to fairly normal adolescence (Bakwin & Bakwin, 1966; Laufer & Denhoff, 1957). Some of the difficulties in assessing outcome for hyperactive children is that the diagnosis has often included many secondary problems such as learning disabilities, aggressiveness, and poor peer interaction, which are known to show considerable continuity into adolescence whether hyperactivity is also present or not. However, there are many studies that clearly attest to a poor outcome for some children who have received a diagnosis of childhood hyperactivity. The most common specific diagnosis in adulthood is *antisocial personality disorder*, which occurred in one quarter of the adults in one followup study of childhood hyperactivity (Weiss et al., 1985). In this study, one half of these children had significant social and psychological problems in adulthood.

Drug Therapy: Hyperactivity

Leaving aside the diagnostic problems related to adolescent hyperactivity, there appears to be a difference in the choice of drugs used for younger and older children. Pfefferbaum and Overall (1984), for example, gave nine clinical descriptions of hypothetical child psychiatric patients to 25 experienced child psychiatrists and asked them to rank order their use of 13 common psychotropic drugs. Two of the vignettes gave clinical descriptions of hyperactivity, with only a difference in age, 6 years versus 15 years. Interestingly, for the 6-year-old child, the psychiatrists ranked the stimulants as the best drug, well above any other medications. For the adolescent, however, Ritalin (methylphenidate) was chosen only a little more often than Mellaril, and Tofranil was selected almost as often as Dexedrine (dextroamphetamine).

These clinical differences probably relate to long-standing beliefs about the limited usefulness and risks associated in treating hyperactive adolescents with stimulants (Safer & Allen, 1975). However, many workers (reviewed by Varley, 1983) have shown that stimulants can produce behavioral and probably academic improvement in selected troubled adolescents with histories of childhood hyperactivity. The proposed problems with growth and potential drug abuse appear minimal at the most. Uncontrolled case reports suggest that even adults with aggressive antisocial personality disorder might benefit from stimulant drug therapy when hyperactivity was present in childhood (Stringer & Josef, 1983). It has also been suggested that certain adults can be identified with a syndrome of restlessness, irritability, depression, and inattentiveness (*Attention Deficit Disorder: Residual Type*) who have early histories of hyperactivity and may benefit from treatment with Ritalin (Wender et al., 1985).

The aforementioned findings need further study and it probably remains true that, in present clinical practice, hyperactive adolescents are likely to receive neuroleptic treatment. The disadvantages of both the stimulants and neuroleptics may lead to further investigation into the benefits of tricyclic medications. Gastfriend et al. (1984), for example, have recently shown a behavioral benefit, similar to reports in childhood, with the tricyclic antidepressant Norpramin (desipramine), in a small group of hyperactive adolescents.

Drug Therapy: Aggression

A number of recent developments have occurred in the pharmacological management of aggression. Normally, aggressive behavior is associated with another well-described disorder, and treatment of the underlying condition is obviously of paramount importance. Aggressive behavior is generally managed with a neuroleptic drug; however, recent interest has focused on tricyclic antidepressants and the stimulants. In the case of intermittent outbursts of violence, three medications (Inderal, lithium, and Tegretol) have shown some early promise of benefit.

Inderal (Propranolol). This drug is largely used medically for cardiac disorders, hypertension, and angina. In psychiatry there has been interest in this drug for treating chronic schizophrenia (Yorkston et al., 1977) and in reducing the physical symptoms of anxiety. Recently, Silver and Yudofsky (1985) listed 10 scientific reports describing 59 patients whose outbursts of rage were controlled to some extent with Inderal. All of the individuals had some form of brain abnormality (seizures, trauma, infections, mental retardation). The drug took between 2 days and 6 weeks to take effect. The dosage required varied considerably, ranging from 50 to 960 mg per day. Side effects included a reduction in blood pressure and pulse rate and rarely breathing difficulties, nightmares, and decreased motor coordination. Because of the potential risks to cardiovascular and respiratory functions and some reports of adverse interactions with neuroleptics, Silver and Yudofsky concluded that under controlled medical circumstances and with caution in using concurrent medication, Inderal is a promising form of treatment for certain types of aggression.

Lithium. Lithium has shown some effectiveness as an antiaggression agent for adolescents and young adults who are mentally retarded and/or have epilepsy as well as for neurologically normal male delinquents (reviewed by Sheard, 1978). Among the latter group, certain characteristics seem to be associated with effectiveness of lithium treatment. These include *mood lability* (rapid changes between euphoria and depression), irritability, hostility, restlessness, impulsivity, and distractibility as well as *pressured speech* (excessive, rapid talking) and loud and provocative manner. Other workers have described a similar personality profile among adolescent females, which they have called the *emotionally unstable character disorder* (Rifkin et al., 1972). This disorder is also purported to show a response to lithium therapy. The dosages of lithium recommended in these studies are the same as those used to control mania in adolescents.

Tegretol (Carbamazepine). There are a number of reports showing that Tegretol is helpful in reducing aggressive and impulsive behavior occurring in patients with a number of different diagnoses, including schizophrenia, personality disorder, and brain disorders such as trauma or seizures (reviewed by Roy-Byrne et al., 1984b). This was not necessarily related to abnormalities detectable on an EEG, which would suggest that the method of action of the drug was not due to its antiepileptic properties. The enthusiasm for Tegretol was tempered by early reports that it might worsen aggression in some children and adolescents, but Roy-Byrne et al. (1984c) have stated that the therapeutic effects of Tegretol are in many ways similar to lithium. This is particularly noticeable in one controlled study that showed that Tegretol significantly reduced self-destructive behavior (overdosing, wrist cutting, and cigarette burning) in 13 females who exhibited symptoms similar to the emotionally unstable character disorder. The dosages of Tegretol used for the control of aggression are the same as those used for the treatment of seizure disorders.

Clinical Suggestions

At this time, there are numerous approaches available to help manage the adolescent with conduct disorder and hyperactivity. The majority of teenagers with antisocial behavior and normal intellect are most likely to benefit from psychosocial interventions or management within the legal system. However, a childhood diagnosis of hyperactivity may suggest benefit from stimulant or tricyclic medication for recurring adolescent difficulties. Severe outbursts of aggression (particularly in combination with neurological disorders) may respond to neuroleptics, but the concerns regarding the long-term use of these medications suggest that Inderal or Tegretol might be more useful drugs to consider. When violent outbursts occur in the presence of a history of mood lability and emotional instability, then consideration should be given to the use of lithium.

DISORDERS OF EATING

Adolescent eating disorders cover a set of largely unique behaviors that begin in this age group, appear to be increasing in incidence, and have achieved considerable notoriety in western society. The two major eating disorders are *anorexia nervosa* and *bulimia*.

The diagnostic criteria for anorexia nervosa and bulimia are presented in Table 5–4 and Table 5–5, respectively. There is considerable overlap between the two disorders, and many females exhibit these behaviors; but they are not always referred for clinical treatment because their eating habits do not create serious problems. Eating disorders occur predominantly in females (9:1) and are generally very secretive behaviors. In anorexic patients, severe emaciation (usually in the presence of a lack of concern) and a high activity level are the characteristic symptoms. Approximately half the anorexic population are strict dieters (often with the aid of diuretics, laxatives, and appetite suppressants), whereas the remaining group share many behavioral and personality characteristics of bulimia. These characteristics include an onset of the disorder in late adolescence (16 to 20 years) and a more extroverted manner with an increase incidence of anxiety, depression, or guilt, as well as impulsiveness, drug and alcohol abuse, stealing, suicide attempts, and self-mutilation. Depressed mood is common with both disorders, and the cyclic mood lability of the bulimic often resembles bipolar affective disorder. Although much of the mood abnormalities may be due to weight fluctuations, there is evidence of a higher incidence of depressive illness and alcoholism in other family members of anorexic and bulimic patients (Hudson et al., 1982, 1983), which suggests that mood disorders might relate to these illnesses.

Drug Therapy

The most common treatments for eating disturbances are psychological, but they are not effective unless close medical supervision of healthy eating habits and appropriate weight gain or stabilization is achieved. Medications that have reportedly shown some benefit during the weight gain phase of anorexia include Thorazine (Dally & Sargant, 1960), tricyclic antidepressants (Needleman and Waber, 1977), Dilantin (Green & Rau, 1977), and an antiasthmatic drug, Periactin (cyproheptadine). Periactin has specific appetite-stimulating properties, and, in combination with the increased weight gain, reduces depressive symptomatology even more rapidly than Elavil (Halmi et al., 1983). Apart from drowsiness, Periactin also seems to have fewer serious side effects than other psychotropic medications. Halmi et al. used a dosage of 32 mg per day, and specific side effects were not reported, although they would be expected to be similar to other antihistamines (e.g., drowsiness, dry mouth, blurred vision,

Table 5–4.   DSM-III Diagnostic Criteria for Anorexia Nervosa[a]

---

1. Intense fear of becoming obese, which does not diminish as weight loss progresses
2. Disturbance of body image (e.g., claiming to "feel fat" even when emaciated)
3. Weight loss of at least 25% of original body weight (or projected body weight if under 18 years old)
4. Refusal to maintain body weight over a minimal normal weight for age and height
5. No known physical illness that would account for the weight loss

---

[a]American Psychiatric Association. (1980). *Diagnostic and statistical manual of mental disorders* (3rd ed.). Washington, DC: Author.

dizziness, nausea, rashes). After weight gain is achieved, most treatment for anorexics is psychotherapeutic in focus, as it is for the bulimics, but long-term management of their behavior problems has shown improvement with the use of tricyclic antidepressants (Pope et al., 1983), MAOIs (Jonas et al., 1983; Walsh et al., 1982), and Dilantin (Green & Rau, 1977; Wermuth et al., 1977). Unfortunately, much of our medical information about the use of these drugs is based upon case studies and excludes a large number of impulsive, self-destructive adolescent bulimics. However, the relationship between bulimia and the emotionally unstable character disorder might explain why 12 out of 14 bulimic patients treated by Hau (1984) showed significant benefit with lithium therapy.

Obesity

Obesity, defined as exceeding ideal weight by 20%, affects as many as 15% of all adolescents. Although there are a number of biological theories of causation, there is not recognized use for medication unless the underlying problem is medically based (e.g., endocrine disorders such as diabetes or thyroid hormone deficiency). In fact, all appetite suppressants are stimulant drugs of some sort, which are potentially drugs of abuse and addiction. Diuretics and laxatives are very dangerous when used in combination with dietary restrictions.

DISORDERS OF EMOTIONS

Emotional disturbance before the onset of puberty is generally characterized as an undifferentiated mixture of anxiety, physical complaints, and *regressed behavior* (reemergence of behavior associated

Table 5–5.   DSM-III Diagnostic Criteria for Bulimia[a]

---

1. Recurrent episodes of binge-eating (rapid consumption of a large amount of food in a discrete period of time, usually less than two hours)
2. At least three of the following:
   a. Consumption of high caloric, easily digested food during a binge
   b. Inconspicuous eating during a binge
   c. Termination of such eating episodes by abdominal pain, sleep, social interruption, or self-induced vomiting
   d. Repeated attempts to lose weight by severely restrictive diets, self-induced vomiting, or use of cathartics or diuretics
   e. Frequent weight fluctuations greater than ten pounds due to alternating binges and fasts
3. Awareness that the eating pattern is abnormal and fear of not being able to stop eating voluntarily.
4. Depressed mood and self-deprecating thoughts following eating binges
5. The bulimic episodes are not due to anorexia nervosa or any other known physical disorder

---

[a]American Psychiatric Association. (1980). *Diagnostic and statistical manual of mental disorders* (3rd ed.). Washington, DC: Author.

with an earlier stage of development), and it often occurs in relation to environmental stresses. The relevance of apparent emotional disturbance can vary with age. Normal fears and anxieties in a young child can appear identical to more serious disorders when seen in an adolescent. A good example of this is observation of a child's reaction to a demand to attend school.

In their first school year, as many as 80% of all children have difficulties with leaving home, of which nearly half are of marked severity. However, most children under 11 years who maintain a reluctance to attend school do not have different attendance patterns from other children. Only a small number of children experience the emotional disorder called *school refusal* (or *school phobia*). Serious cases of school refusal are often characterized by poor school attainment, an anxious home environment, more frequent physical complaints, and an abnormal overdependent mother-child relationship. Predisposition to such problems may also be due to individual variation in personality style and possible susceptibility to mood disturbance or phobic states.

The implication from this one example is seen in other emotional disorders of childhood. It appears that a large number of children experience appropriate anxiety about strange events and people as well as a natural development of certain types of fears (e.g., animals, abandonment, parents' health). However, by adolescence, continuing emotional disorders are often related to familial, constitutional, and environmental factors and begin to differentiate into the more classical group of anxiety disorders described in adult psychiatry.

Anxiety States

The three major groups of anxiety disorders are generalized anxiety disorder, panic disorder, and obsessive-compulsive disorder. The symptoms of each are briefly presented here.

Generalized Anxiety Disorder. This disorder is defined as a chronic (at least 1 month) disabling sense of anxiety, usually characterized by shakiness, jitteriness, fidgeting, apprehensiveness, and extreme watchfulness. Its physical symptoms may include a raised pulse rate, gastric or intestinal complaints, and tremor. The symptoms are always present and are *not* related to any particular stressor (e.g., taking academic exams).

Panic Disorder. Recurrent, spontaneous sudden episodes of fear, apprehension, or feelings of impending doom are referred to as panic disorders. Panic attack symptoms include difficulty breathing, palpitations (heart beating hard and/or fast), chest pain, choking, dizziness, feelings of unreality, numbness in limbs, sweating, and faintness. There is often a feeling that one may die, go crazy, or lose control.

Obsessive-Compulsive Disorder. There is evidence that at least some individuals with obsessive-compulsive disorder have a chronic neurobiologic disturbance, often with a waxing and waning of symptomatology during their entire life-cycle. Obsessive-compulsive symptoms may also occur at some time during the course of schizophrenic, manic, or depressive illness and remit with appropriate treatment of the primary disorder. *Obsessions* are recurrent ideas, thoughts, images, or internal impulses that incessantly come to the level of consciousness and seem senseless or even distasteful to the person. Obsessions can be extremely varied and range from simple (e.g., impulse to count numbers in one's head, repeat words or phrases) to more complex mental activities. They may be related to fears of harm, infestation, or loss of self-control. Commonly, these obsessional thoughts are associated with ritualistic physical acts, such as repetitive washing, arrangement of objects, or movements of the body, which are collectively referred to as *compulsions*.

Phobic Disorders

Disorders in which fear and avoidance of a certain object or situation leads to restriction of normal activities are called *phobic disorders*. There are three general types: agoraphobia, social phobia, and simple phobia.

Agoraphobia. A fear of being in public places and crowds and paradoxically often a fear of being alone are the major features of agoraphobia. Panic attacks commonly occur in this condition.

Social Phobia. Avoidance of, or anxiety in, social situations due to an irrational fear of behaving in an embarrassing or humiliating manner is referred to as social phobia.

Simple Phobia. Incapacitating fears to specific objects or animals, such as dogs or spiders, are called simple phobias.

Post-traumatic Stress Disorder

Severe distressing events such as accidents or natural disasters or extremely threatening situations can be followed by an immediate or delayed pathological reaction characterized by reexperiencing the event through nightmares or sudden vivid recollection. This reaction, referred to as posttraumatic stress disorder, is sometimes associated with emotional numbing, a limited range of mood, and apparent detachment. Alternatively, there is excessive vigilance and an exaggerated startle response to minor events. Insomnia is common.

General Comments

Panic disorder, obsessive-compulsive disorder, and social phobias commonly have their onset in adolescence, but all of the aforementioned disorders can occur during this stage of development. Unfortunately, emotional disorders of adolescents are usually chronic in nature. There is undoubtedly some overlap between anxiety disorders and depression in certain patients, and milder depressed states may have a predominance of anxiety symptoms.

Interestingly, there is relationship between school phobia (or refusal) and (adult) agoraphobia. Both are associated with panic attacks, and their victims stay home excessively, often requiring the support of family or a close friend to go into certain situations. Berg (1981) reviewed the literature on school refusers, and there is evidence that a significant number of adult agoraphobics were school refusers in earlier years and that daughters of agoraphobic mothers are at higher risk to develop school phobia.

Because adolescent anxiety disorders are similar to adult states, it is reasonable to use the experience of adult psychiatrists in management of emotional disorders (reviewed by Brown et al., 1984). This is helpful because only with school phobia has there been any significant adolescent studies on the value of drug treatment. Some of the major advances in treatment of anxiety and phobias have been in the area of behavior therapy, which challenges the thinking patterns of the patient and incorporates relaxation techniques with internal imagery of fears and/or direct exposure to fears.

Drug Therapy

Drugs that have been found to be useful in the treatment of emotional disorders are Inderal, MAOIs, tricyclic antidepressants, and specific antianxiety drugs: the benzodiazepines (e.g., Valium, Librium).

Inderal (propranolol) has been known to reduce the physical symptoms of anxiety since the 1960s, but controlled studies of the different anxiety disorders have produced discrepant results. Some clinicians suggest that Inderal is comparable with the benzodiazepines and (given fears about the dependency and abuse of the latter) may be a useful adjunct therapy. Clinical experience suggests that although Inderal may block the physical aspects of anxiety, the perception of fear is unchanged, unlike most benzodiazepines, which also have a central calming effect.

The benzodiazepines (Valium and Librium) have dominated the market for management of anxiety symptoms, and the level of drug prescribing by the late 1970s had reached staggering proportions. Until then, these drugs were considered safe (even in very large doses), and the major complications were related to sedation and reduced coordination. Occasionally, a "paradoxical reaction" occurred when susceptible individuals became aggressive and hostile. However, concerns about the level of prescribing, the tendency to use the drugs to avoid more active psychological therapies, and reports of abuse and even physiological addiction has led to a reappraisal of their use.

At this time, short-term drug therapy (2 to 3 months) for anxiety states while initiating psychological treatments seems to be the most common clinical practice. Many practitioners are using the more rapidly eliminated benzodiazepines, such as Ativan (lorazepam) or Xanax (alprazolam), but it is uncertain if this is of significant clinical advantage. Inderal and the benzodiazepines have been indicated for most anxiety states except obsessive-compulsive disorder.

The two antidepressant treatments (tricyclics and MAOIs) have shown some specific benefits for agoraphobia, panic disorder, and obsessive-compulsive disorder. One particular researcher has been interested in the usefulness of tricyclic antidepressants for the treatment of panic attacks in agoraphobic patients (Klein, 1981). His early work has generally been confirmed, and it was extended to the syndrome of school phobia (Gittelman-Klein & Klein, 1971). In a well-controlled study of 35 school phobic children, there was considerable reduction in depression, severity of phobia, maternal dependence, physical complaints, and fear of going to school following treatment with Tofranil in doses ranging from 100 to 200 mg per day. British workers are less enthusiastic about this type of medication and have shown that behavioral treatments can be as effective in treatment of agoraphobia (Marks et al., 1983) and school phobia (Berney et al., 1981).

The tricyclic, Anafranil (clomipramine), presently unavailable in the United States, is of interest in the treatment of anxiety states because it has been shown to be an effective agent in some individuals with obsessive-compulsive disorder (reviewed by Elkins et al., 1980). Other drugs, including the MAOIs, have also been reported to benefit obsessional states in uncontrolled studies. the MAOIs are useful for the treatment of panic attacks and may even be superior to tricyclics (Sheehan et al., 1980), but concerns about their safety prevent the general acceptance of them as the drug of first choice.

GENERAL ISSUES ABOUT DRUG THERAPY IN ADOLESCENTS

This chapter has addressed the classical syndromes seen in adolescent psychiatry and the drugs that are generally used in their management. This does not, however, exhaust all the clinical psychiatric situations in which drug therapy or drug interactions may be of importance (e.g., sleep disorders, enuresis, encopresis, drug and alcohol abuse). Perhaps the most difficult situation is in helping adolescents who have a physical illness in combination with psychological problems.

Chronic illness with or without additional physical handicaps can be a difficult situation to manage at any age. However, the importance of physical appearance and peer acceptance during adolescence can make physical illness a very traumatic and, at times, self-destructive experience. The psychiatrist's role is in helping the adolescent adjust to the effects and demands of managing their illness. Depressive reactions can be quite common in these situations, often manifested with anger and hostility, but the psychiatrist must also be aware of the potential psychological reactions to the treatment itself or directly caused by it. For example, steroid drug treatment (hormone therapy), commonly used in the treatment of immunological disorders, can cause severe psychological change, usually mimicking depression or mania.

This example highlights the problems the psychiatrist faces when treating adolescents. Psychological problems can be extreme and volatile, and the causes are often multifaceted. In other words, many different elements (biological, psychological, and environmental) interact to produce a psychiatric disorder. For this reason, different types of intervention might produce some improvement for the adolescent, but the social and personal pressures on the psychiatrist to successfully and rapidly "treat" the adolescent can lead to the use of drugs before other treatment approaches have been tried.

Ideally, drug treatment would only be used for adolescent psychiatric disorders in which a biological disturbance is being specifically improved by the action of the drug itself. Many of the descriptions of drug use in this chapter have shown that although medication may improve target symptoms, it does not necessarily alter the overall course of illness. It is important, therefore, that the risks of drug therapy are clearly weighed against the benefits. It is not unusual for the side effects of a particular drug to lead to additional medications to manage the side effects (for example, the concomitant use of anticholinergic and neuroleptic drugs). For the severely disturbed adolescent, the necessity for such treatment may be appropriate. However, the addition of tricyclic medication to treat drug-induced school phobia in children and adolescents receiving neuroleptic medication for Tourette syndrome creates a worrying precedent (Linet, 1985).

In summary, therefore, it is important to realize the limitations of our present drug armamentarium as well as the benefits. Pharmacotherapy can, at times, be crucial to recovery, but even in disorders such as major depression, in which the benefit of antidepressant medication seems convincing, secondary social handicaps may remain after recovery and will require more intensive psychological therapies (Puig-Antich et al., 1985). The majority of adolescent disorders respond to psychological interventions without medication and except in rare circumstances, such as acute psychosis, these interventions are the generally recommended first appraoch.

SUGGESTED READINGS

Anthony, E. J. (1982). Normal adolescent development from a cognitive viewpoint. *Journal of the American Academy of Child Psychiatry, 21,* 318–327. (C)

Berg, I. (1984). Reading about adolescence. *British Journal of Psychiatry,* 144, 94–97. (C, P, S)

Brown, J. T., Mulrow, C. D., & Stoudemire, G. A. (1984). The anxiety disorders. *Annals of Internal Medicine, 100,* 558–564. (C)

Erikson, E. H. (1968). *Identity, youth and crisis.* New York: Norton. (C, S)

Gualtieri, C. T., Barnhill, J., McGinsey, J., & Schell, D. (1980). Tardive dyskinesia and other movement disorders in children treated with psychotropic drugs. *Journal of the American Academy of Child Psychiatry, 19,* 491–510. (C)

Pharmacotherapy for ADD-H adolescent workshop. (1985). *Psychopharmacology Bulletin, 21,* 169–257. (C, S)

Rutter, M. (1980). *Changing youth in a changing society.* Cambridge: Harvard University Press. (C, S)

Steinberg, D. (1981). The use of lithium carbonate in adolescence. *Journal of Child Psychology and Psychiatry, 21,* 263–271. (C)

REFERENCES

American Psychiatric Association. (1980). *Diagnostic and statistical manual of mental disorders* (3rd ed.). Washington, DC: Author.

Andreason, N. C., & Hoenk, P. R. (1982). The predictive value of adjustment disorder: A follow-up study. *American Journal of Psychiatry, 130,* 585–590.

Anthony, E. J. (1982). Normal adolescent development from a cognitive viewpoint. *Journal of the American Academy of Child Psychiatry, 21,* 318–327.

Apter, A., Dickerman, Z., Gonen, N., Assa, S., Prager-Lewin, R., Kaufman, H., Tyano, S., & Laroy, Z. (1983). The effect of chlorpromazine on hypothalamic-pituitary-gonadal function in 10 adolescent schizophrenic boys. *American Journal of Psychiatry, 140,* 1588–1591.

Bakwin, H., & Bakwin, R. (1966). *Clinical management of behavior disorders in children.* Philadelphia: W. B. Saunders.

Bakwin, H. (1957). Suicide in children and adolescents. *Journal of Pediatrics, 50,* 749–769.

Baldessarini, R. J. (1980). Drugs and the treatment of psychiatric disorders. In A. G. Gilman, L. S. Goodman, & A. Gilman (Eds.), *The pharmacological basis of therapeutics* (6th ed., pp. 391–447). New York: Macmillan.

Ballenger, J. C., & Post, R. M. (1978). Therapeutic effects of carbamazepine in affective illness; a preliminary report. *Communication in Psychopharmacology, 2,* 159–175.

Baltes, P., & Nesselroade, J. (1972). Cultural change and adolescent personality development: An application of longitudinal sequences. *Developmental Psychology, 7,* 244–256.

Bengston, V., & Starr, J. (1975). Contrast and consensus: A generational analysis of youth in the 1970s. In T. Havighurst & P. Dryer (Eds.), *Youth.* Chicago: University of Chicago Press.

Berg, I. (1981). When truants and school refusers grow up. *British Journal of Psychiatry, 141,* 208–210.

Berg, I. (1984). Reading about adolescence. *British Journal of Psychiatry, 144,* 94–97.

Berney, T. B., Kolvin, I., Bhate, S. R., Garside, R. F., Jeans, J., Kay, B., & Scarth, L. (1981). School phobia: A therapeutic trial with clomipramine and outcome. *British Journal of Psychiatry, 138,* 110–118.

Blos, P. (1970). *The young adolescent: Clinical studies.* London: Collier-Macmillan.

Braungart, R. C. (1975). Youth and social movements. In S. E. Dragastin & G. H. Elder (Eds.), *Adolescence in the life cycle: Psychological change and social content.* London: Halsted Press.

Brown, J. T., Mulrow, C. D., & Stoudemire, G. A. (1984). The anxiety disorders. *Annals of Internal Medicine, 100,* 558–564.

Campbell, M., Schulman, D., & Rapoport, J. L. (1978). The current status of lithium therapy in child and adolescent psychiatry. *Journal of American Academy of Child Psychiatry, 17,* 717–720.

Capes, M., Gould, E., & Townsend, M. (1971). *Stress in youth.* London: Oxford University Press.

Carr, V., Dorrington, C., Schrader, G., & Wade, J. (1983). The use of ECT for mania in childhood bipolar disorder. *British Journal of Psychiatry, 143,* 411–415.

Dally, P. J., & Sargant, W. (1960). A new treatment of anorexia nervosa. *British Medical Journal, 1,* 1770–1773.

Elkins, R., Rapoport, J. L., & Lynsley, A. (1980). Obsessive-compulsive disorder of childhood and adolescence. A neurobiologic viewpoint. *Journal of the American Academy of Child Psychiatry, 19,* 511–524.

Erickson, W. D., Yellin, A. M., Hopwood, J. H., Realmuto, G. M., & Greenberg, L. M. (1984). The effects of neuroleptics on attention in adolescent schizophrenics. *Biological Psychiatry, 19,* 745–753.

Erikson, E. H. (1968). *Identity, youth and crisis.* New York: Norton.

Esman, A. H. (1981). Appropriate use of psychotropics in adolescents. *Hospital,* 49–60.

Farrington, D. (1978). The family background of aggressive youths. In L. Hersov, M. Berger, & D. Shaffer (Eds.), *Aggression and antisocial behaviour in childhood and adolescence* (pp. 73–93). Oxford: Pergamon.

Freud, A. (1958). Adolescence. *Psychoanalytic study of the child, 13,* 255–278.

Gastfriend, D. R., Biederman, J., & Jellinek, M. S. (1984). Desipramine in the treatment of adolescents with attention deficit disorder. *American Journal of Psychiatry, 141,* 906–908.

Gittelman-Klein, R., & Klein, D. F. (1971). Controlled imipramine treatment of school phobia. *Archives of General Psychiatry, 25,* 204–207.

Goodenough, F. L. (1931). *Anger in young children.* Minneapolis: University of Minnesota Press.

Graham, P., & Rutter, M. (1973). Psychiatric disorder in the young adolescent: A follow-up study. *Proceedings of the Royal Society of Medicine, 66,* 1226–1229.

Green, R. S., & Rau, J. H. (1977). The use of diphenylhydantoin in compulsive eating disorder: Further studies. In R. A. Vigersky (Ed.), *Anorexia nervosa* (pp. 377–382). New York: Raven Press.

Gualtieri, C. T., Barnhill, J., McGinsey, J., & Schell, D. (1980). Tardive dyskinesia and other movement disorders in children treated with psychotropic drugs. *Journal of the American Academy of Child Psychiatry, 19,* 491–510.

Gualtieri, C. T., Quade, D., Hicks, R. E., Mayo, J. P., & Schroeder, S. R. (1984). Tardive dyskinesia and other clinical consequences of neuroleptic treatment in children and adolescents. *American Journal of Psychiatry, 141,* 20–23.

Hall, G. S. (1904). *Adolescence: Its psychology and its relation to physiology, anthropology, sociology, sex, crime, religion and education.* New York: Appelton.

Halmi, K. A., Eckert, E., & Falk, J. R. (1983). Cyproheptadine, an antidepressant and weight inducing drug for anorexia nervosa. *Psychopharmacology Bulletin, 19,* 103–105.

Hassanyeh, F., & Davidson, K. (1980). Bipolar affective psychosis with onset before age 16 years. Report of 10 cases. *British Journal of Psychiatry, 137,* 530–539.

Hsu, L. G. G. (1984). Treatment of bulimia with lithium. *American Journal of Psychiatry, 141,* 1260–1262.

Hudson, J. I., Laffer, P. S., & Pope, H. G. (1982). Bulimia related to affective disorder by family history and response to dexamethasone suppression test. *American Journal of Psychiatry, 139,* 685–687.

Hudson, J. I., Pope, H. G., Jonas, J. M., & Yurgelun-Todd, D. (1983). Family history study of anorexia nervosa and bulimia. *British Journal of Psychiatry, 142,* 133–138.

Inhelder, B., & Piaget, J. (1958). *The growth of logical thinking from childhood to adolescence* (translated by A. Parson and S. Milgram). New York: Basic Books.

Jonas, J. M., Hudson, J. I., & Pope, H. G. (1983). Treatment of bulimia with monoamine oxidase inhibitors. *Journal of Clinical Psychopharmacology, 3,* 59–60.

Kagan, J., & Moss, H. (1962). *From birth to maturity.* New York: Wiley.

Kishimoto, A., Ogura, C., Hazama, H., & Inoue, K. (1983). Long-term prophylactic effects of carbamazepine in affective disorder. *British Journal of Psychiatry, 143,* 327–331.

Klein, D. F. (1981). Anxiety reconceptualized. In D. F. Klein & J. G. Rabkin (Eds.), *Anxiety: New research and current concepts.* New York: Raven Press.

Laufer, M., & Denhoff, E. (1957). Hyperkinetic behavior disorders in childhood. *Journal of Pediatrics, 50,* 463–474.

Linet, L. S. (1985). Tourette syndrome, pimozide and school phobia: The neuroleptic separation anxiety syndrome. *American Journal of Psychiatry, 142,* 613–615.

Manning, M., Heron, J., & Marshall, T. (1978). Styles of hostility and social interactions at nursery, at school and at home. In L. Hersov, M. Berger, & D. Shaffer (Eds.), *Aggression and antisocial behaviour in childhood and adolescence* (pp. 29–58). Oxford: Pergamon.

Marks, I. M., Gray, S., Cohen, D., Hill, R., Mawson, D., Ramm, E., & Stern, R. S. (1983). Imipramine and brief therapist-aided exposure in agoraphobics having self-exposure homework. *Archives of General Psychiatry, 40,* 153–162.

Masterson, J. F. (1967). The symptomatic adolescent five years later. He didn't grow out of it. *American Journal of Psychiatry, 123,* 1338–1345.

Needleman, H., & Waber, D. (1977). The use of amitriptyline in anorexia nervosa. In R. A. Vigersky (Ed.), *Anorexia nervosa* (pp. 357–362). New York: Raven Books.

Offer, D., & Offer, J. (1975). *From teenage to young manhood.* New York: Basic Books.

Pfefferbaum, B., & Overall, J. F. (1984). Decisions about drug treatment in children. *Journal of the American Academy of Child Psychiatry, 23,* 209–214.

Pope, H. G., Hudson, J. I., Jonas, J. M., & Yurgelun-Todd, D. (1983). Bulimia treated with imipramine: A placebo-controlled, double-blind study. *American Journal of Psychiatry, 140,* 554–558.

Puig-Antich, J., Luhens, E., Davies, M., Goetz, D., Brennan-Quattrock, J., & Todak, G. (1985). Psychosocial functioning in prepubertal major depressive disorders. II. Interpersonal relationships after sustained recovery from affective episode. *Archives of General Psychiatry, 42,* 511–517.

Quinn, P., & Rapoport, J. (1975). One year follow-up of hyperactive boys treated with imipramine or methylphenidate. *American Journal of Psychiatry, 132,* 241–245.

Rapoport, J., Quinn, P., Bradbard, G., Riddle, D., & Brooks, E. (1974). Imipramine and methylphenidate treatments of hyperactive boys: A double-blind comparison. *Archives of General Psychiatry, 30,* 789–793.

Realmuto, G. M., Erickson, W. D., Yellin, A. M., Hopwood, J. H., & Greenberg, L. M. (1984). Clinical comparison of thiothixene and thioridazine in schizophrenic adolescents. *American Journal of Psychiatry, 141,* 440–442.

Rifkin, A., Quitkin, F., Carillo, C., Blumberg, A. G., & Klein, D. F. (1972). Lithium carbonate in emotionally unstable character disorder. *Archives of General Psychiatry, 27,* 519–523.

Rosen, B. M., Bahn, A. K., Shellow, R., & Bower, E. M. (1965). Adolescent patients served in outpatient psychiatric clinics. *American Journal of Public Health, 55,* 1563–1577.

Roy-Byrne, P. P., Joffe, R. T., Uhde, T. W., & Post, R. M. (1984a). Approaches to the evaluation and treatment of rapid-cycling affective illness. *British Journal of Psychiatry, 145,* 543–550.

Roy-Byrne, P. P., Uhde, T. W., & Post, R. M. (1984b). Carbamazepine for aggression, schizophrenia and nonaffective syndromes. *International Drug Therapy Newsletter, 19,* 9–12.

Boy-Byrne, P. P., Uhde, T. W., & Post, R. M. (1984c). Carbamazepine for hyperactivity, anxiety and withdrawal syndromes. *International Drug Therapy Newsletter, 19,* 25–26.

Rutter, M. (1980). *Changing youth in a changing society.* Cambridge: Harvard University Press.

Rutter, M., Graham, P., Chadwick, O., & Yule, W. (1976). Adolescent turmoil: Fact or fiction. *Journal of Child Psychology and Psychiatry, 17,* 35–36.

Safer, D., & Allen, R. (1975). Stimulant drug treatment of hyperactive adolescents. *Diseases of the Nervous System, 368,* 454–457.

Sheard, M. H. (1978). The effect of lithium and other ions on aggressive behavior. In L. Valzelli (Ed.), *Modern problems of pharmacopsychiatry* (Vol. 13, pp. 53–68). New York: Karger.

Sheehan, D. V., Ballenger, J., & Jacobsen, G. (1980). Treatment of endogenous anxiety with phobic, hysterical and hypochondrial symptoms. *Archives of General Psychiatry, 37*, 51–59.

Shukla, S, Godwin, C. D., Long, L. E. B., & Miller, M. (1984). Lithium-carbamazepine neurotoxicity and risk factors. *American Journal of Psychiatry, 141*, 1604–1606.

Silver, J. M., & Yudofsky, S. (1985). Propranolol for aggression: Literature review and clinical guidelines. *International Drug Therapy Newsletter, 20*, 9–12.

Steinberg, D. (1980). The use of lithium carbonate in adolescence. *Journal of Child Psychology and Psychiatry, 21*, 263–271.

Stringer, A. Y., & Josef, N. D. (1983). Methylphenidate in the treatment of aggression in two patients with antisocial personality disorder. *American Journal of Psychiatry, 140*, 1365–1366.

Varley, C. K. (1983). Effects of methylphenidate in adolescents with attention deficit disorder. *Journal of the American Academy of Child Psychiatry, 24*, 351–354.

Walsh, B. T., Stewart, J. W., Wright, L., Harrison, W., Roose, S. P., & Glassman, A. H. (1982). Treatment of bulimia with monoamine oxidase inhibition. *American Journal of Psychiatry, 139*, 1629–1630.

Warneke, L. (1975). A case of manic-depressive illness in childhood. *Canadian Psychiatric Association Journal, 20*, 195–200.

Wender, P. H., Reimherr, F. W., Wood, D., & Ward, M. (1985). A controlled study of methylphenidate in the treatment of attention deficit disorder, residual type, in adults. *American Journal of Psychiatry, 142*, 547–552.

Weinberg, W. A., & Brumback, R. A. (1976). Mania in childhood. Case studies and literature review. *American Journal of Diseases of Children, 130*, 380–385.

Weiner, I. B., & Del Gaudio, A. C. (1976). Psychopathology in adolescence. An epidemiological study. *Archives of General Psychiatry, 33*, 187–193.

Weiss, G., Hechtman, L., Milroy, T., & Perlman, T. (1985). Psychiatric status of hyperactives as adults: A controlled prospective 15-year follow-up of 63 hyperactive children. *Journal of the American Academy of Child Psychiatry, 24*, 211–220.

Welner, A., Welner, Z., & Fishman, R. (1979). Psychiatric adolescent inpatients: Eight to ten year follow-up. *Archives of General Psychiatry, 36*, 698–700.

Wermuth, B. M., Davis, K. L., Hollister, L. E., & Stunkard, A. J. (1977). Phenytoin treatment of the binge-eating syndrome. *American Journal of Psychiatry, 134*, 1249–1253.

Yepes, L., Balka, E., Winsberg, B., & Bialer, I. (1977). Amitriptyline and methylphenidate treatment of behaviorally disordered children. *Journal of Child Psychology and Psychiatry, 18*, 39–52.

Yorkston, N. Z., Gruzelier, J. H., Zaki, S. A., Hollander, D., Pitcher, D., & Sergeant, H. S. (1977). Propranolol as an adjunct to the treatment of schizophrenia. *Lancet, 1*, 575–578.

Youngerman, J., & Canino, I. A. (1978). Lithium carbonate use in children and adults. *Archives of General Psychiatry, 35*, 216–224.

Chapter 6

Other Disorders

Psychotropic drugs are prescribed for a variety of other conditions, which, due either to their rarity or to the use of medication for severe cases only, can be considered uncommon, at least in comparison with certain psychiatric or seizure disorders. Several of these conditions are discussed in this chapter. They are presented in alphabetical order and include the following: cerebral palsy, enuresis, separation anxiety (school phobia), and Tourette syndrome. The general pattern of discussion is a description of the symptoms, the prevalance of the disorder and the use of medication (if known), pharmacotherapy, and in some instances nondrug treatments. The primary focus is on treatment characteristics for elementary school–aged children.

CEREBRAL PALSY

Cerebral palsy refers to a variety of nonprogressive conditions characterized by impairment of motor control, which is the result of damage to the motor areas of the brain either before, during, or soon after the child is born. A number of factors can produce this damage including prenatal diseases, lack of oxygen at birth, and other birth injuries. Approximately 0.3% of the school-aged chilren in the United States have cerebral palsy (Baker, 1959). Mental retardation is common; over half of the children with cerebral palsy score 70 or below on standardized IQ tests. It is noteworthy that accurate assessment of IQ in children with cerebral palsy can be quite difficult, especially if the condition is marked by severe sensory or motor impairment. Many of these children are served in special classes for mentally retarded, physically (orthopedically) impaired, or multiply handicapped students. However, the recent emphasis on least restrictive placement is bringing children with cerebral palsy into the mainstream of school activities. The motor disorders that are collectively called cerebral palsy can be subdivided into several categories, one of which (spasticity) is pertinent to this discussion.

Neural impulses are continually transmitted from the brain to the skeletal muscles via the spinal cord. This creates a slight amount of tension (*muscle tone*), which keeps the muscle taut so it can react to stimuli more quickly. Damage to a certain area of the brain impairs normal motor control, resulting in an excessive amount of muscle tension (*hypertonicity*). This condition is referred to as *spasticity*. It primarily affects the muscles responsible for bending a joint (flexor muscles) as opposed to muscles responsible for extending a joint (extensor muscles). Even slight stimulation causes the muscle to contract, making the person very rigid. Motor movements are slow and spasmodic, and reflexes are often exaggerated. Deliberate efforts to control motor movements usually make things worse because the muscles tighten and become even more spastic. Spasticity is present in approximately half of the children with cerebral palsy and is more apt to be associated with mental retardation than are the other varieties of this disorder.

Behavior disorders (primarily hyperactivity) and epilepsy are frequently associated with cerebral palsy. The prevalence rates for seizure disorders range from 30 to 40% in this population (Cruickshank & Raus, 1955). The relationship between IQ and epilepsy is striking. One survey of individuals with cerebral palsy reported that 72% of those who were mentally retarded (IQ below 70) had epilepsy, compared with 8% in the low normal range (IQ between 85 and 99) (Dunsdon, 1952).

Drug Therapy

The skeletal muscle relaxants are the most commonly prescribed drugs for the symptoms associated with cerebral palsy and are used to treat spasticity. It must be emphasized that spasticity in any particular individual can be the product of one or more different physiological mechanisms and that the various antispasticity drugs affect the body in different ways (see McLellan, 1983). Historically, the most significant early drug discoveries were Antodyne (noxypropanediol) in 1910 and mephenesin in 1949 (Domino, 1974). These agents were desirable because they did not produce sedation; but, unfortunately, they were eventually proven to be of little value at tolerable dosage levels. People have also observed for some time the beneficial effects of alcoholic beverages. Perlstein (1955) noted that alcohol "shows the greatest specific effect. . . .in reducing tensions in cerebral palsy. . . .Many patients can walk with increasing steadiness or write a more legible letter after a cocktail" (p. 239).

It was not until the 1950s, with the development of antianxiety agents, that useable drugs became available. Both the propanediols (Miltown, Equanil) and benzodiazepines (Librium, Valium) are centrally acting skeletal muscle relaxants that benefit some people with cerebral palsy. Although Valium (diazepam) is still used with some frequency, much work remains to be done in this area. Domino (1974) observed that Valium "is of limited value as a skeletal-muscle relaxant because it is a sedative and it is weak, even though it is clearly one of the most useful agents now available" (p. 372). The dose of Valium for children ranges from 6 to 15 mg per day, which is administered in three divided doses (Kendall, 1964). The most common side effects are lethargy, drowsiness, depression, ataxia, nausea, vomiting, and vertigo.

Dantrium (dantrolene sodium), a more recently approved (1974) skeletal muscle relaxant, has been shown to be better than placebo in treating spasticity (Denhoff et al., 1975). The daily dose employed by Denhoff et al. was 12 mg/kg per day divided into four doses. The peak effect of one oral dose occurs about 3 hours after ingestion. The side effects they reported were irritability, lethargy, drowsiness, and general *malaise*. All were transient, disappearing within a week. After the study was completed (6 weeks on medication), nine children were kept on Dantrium. Of these, four showed an increase in seizures (all were epileptic). Therefore, it was concluded that this drug may lower the seizure threshold in some children. Because there is a risk of liver toxicity at dosages above 400 mg per day, liver function tests should be routinely administered when high dosages are used (McLellan, 1983). Mild abnormalities in liver function are indicated by these tests in approximately 10% of patients after the onset of treatment, but they usually abate as treatment progresses. The drug should be gradually discontinued if there is no benefit after 6 weeks of treatment (Roberts & Wright, 1983).

Very little survey data are available on the prevalence of drug therapy for spasticity among children who have cerebral palsy. In one study of 3,306 children in trainable mentally retarded (TMR) programs, it was reported that 22 youngsters received muscle relaxants for cerebral palsy (Gadow & Kalachnik, 1981). The most frequently prescribed drugs were Valium and Dantrium.

It is often difficult to demonstrate benefit from muscle relaxants in people with cerebral palsy, due to measurement problems. Also, there is often a powerful placebo response in studies involving this population. The importance of data based procedures for evaluating the effects of muscle relaxants in habilitative settings has been advocated for some time (Phelps, 1964).

ENURESIS

Nocturnal enuresis refers to involuntary bedwetting during sleep. The disorder is relatively common, affecting about 15% of the physically and mentally normal children at 6 years of age (Azrin & Thienes, 1978). There are, however, cross-cultural differences in the prevalence of enuresis. The rate for the United Kingdom, for example, is lower than the rate for the United States. From age 6 to 20 years, there is a decline in the prevalence of enuresis, with few people bedwetting after 20 years of age. Enuresis is usually not considered a problem until a child is of school age. Clinicians have arbitrarily decided that by the time a child is 6 years old something should be done (Werry, 1965). Enuresis is not usually associated with organic pathology (Forsythe & Redmond, 1974), and psychopathology is negligible (Werry, 1965). If left untreated, there is usually a spontaneous remission of symptoms (the problem seems to cure itself). A distinction is made between children who have never achieved bladder control (primary enuresis) and children who have been "dry" for at least 6 months and then start to wet the bed again (secondary enuresis). There does not, however, appear to be a difference in these two types of enuresis as far as responsiveness to treatment or probability of relapse.

Drug Therapy

In an excellent review of the literature, Blackwell and Currah (1972) stated that the tricyclic antidepressants are the only drugs that have consistently proved to be more effective than placebo for the treatment of nocturnal enuresis. Several different tricyclics are presently available, but Tofranil (imipramine) is the most commonly used for this disorder. It was first reported effective for the treatment of enuresis by MacLean in 1960 and 13 years later was approved by the (FDA) Food and Drug Administration in the United States for use with this disorder. Other tricyclics used for enuresis include Norpramin or Pertofrane (both are desipramine) and Elavil (amitriptyline).

When Tofranil works, the response is immediate, usually during the first week of treatment. A complete cure (total remission of symptoms), however, is reported for less than half of the children on medication. It should be noted that if a less stringent criterion is used (e.g., 50% fewer wet nights), the "success" rate is much higher. Unfortunately, "relapse tends to occur immediately following withdrawal after short periods of treatment, and long-term followup studies suggest that total remission (no wet nights) occurs in only a minority of patients" (Blackwell & Currah, 1972, p. 253).

The total daily dose of Tofranil commonly reported in the literature is 25 to 50 mg given in one oral dose at bedtime. For children over 12 years of age, the dose may be increased to 75 mg if the smaller amount is unsuccessful. The FDA recommends that the dose of Tofranil not exceed 2.5 mg/kg per day because there is a risk of severe side effects at higher doses (Robison & Barker, 1976).

The side effects encountered with Tofranil at doses used for enuresis are usually minor, and children often develop a tolerance for those that do occur. The most common adverse reactions are nervousness, lethargy, drowsiness, and nausea. Abrupt cessation of medication may produce withdrawal symptoms such as nausea and headache. One of the more serious side effects is an adverse effect on the heart (cardiotoxic) at high doses (Robison & Barker, 1976). It is for this reason that low doses (2.5 mg/kg per day or less) are recommended for enuresis. Special care should be given to storing Tofranil out of the reach of children. In the United Kingdom, tricyclic antidepressants are the most common cause of death in children due to accidental poisoning (Cronin et al., 1979). Typically, the drug was prescribed for an adult, either parent or neighbor, for a psychiatric disorder (Parkin & Fraser, 1972). However, in over a fourth of the hospital admissions due to tricyclic poisoning, the drug was prescribed for the treatment of enuresis, often to children under 5 years of age. Therefore, childproof containers are mandatory when prescribing for young patients or for adults with small children.

Day wetting is referred to as *diurnal enuresis*. This condition is more common in females and is often associated with behavior problems at home and at school (Meadow & Berg, 1982). It is a difficult disorder to treat successfully (i.e., no relapses). In one study that examined the utility of two different dosages of Tofranil (25 mg and 50 mg administered in the morning) for diurnal enuresis, Meadow and Berg (1982) found that medication was *not* more effective than placebo.

Although stimulant drugs are not generally used for treating nocturnal enuresis, there have been numerous reports over the years of how hyperactive children with nocturnal enuresis became dry after taking stimulant medication for hyperactivity. Research on stimulants for enuresis has a long history (e.g., Molitch & Poliakoff, 1937). It has recently been suggested that stimulant medication (Ritalin) may be an effective treatment for secondary enuresis (Diamond & Stein, 1983), but Blackwell and Currah (1972) concluded after reviewing the medical literature that the tricyclics were generally more effective.

Nondrug Therapy

A method that is considered by some to be more effective for enuresis than drug therapy is a battery-operated buzzer and pad device, which is quite safe (Meadow, 1977; Stewart, 1975). This method was first developed at the beginning of the century. A 1905 patent describes a buzzer-pad device for which the following claim was made (Mountjoy et al., 1984):

> On the sounding of the alarm the wearer is at once awakened, and in the course of time the habit of awakening as soon as any desire of emission is felt will be established. (p. 301)

This procedure did not become popular, however, until the late 1930s when Mowrer (1938) published a description of his bed-wetting device. The child sleeps on a pad containing two foil electrodes. When a small amount of urine wets the pad, the circuit is closed, triggering an alarm that awakens the sleeping child. In principle, bladder distention becomes associated with awakening and with contraction of the bladder sphincter muscle. In time, the reflex to urinate during sleep is replaced with conditioned bladder control and an increased capacity to retain more urine without awakening (Mowrer, 1950; Stewart, 1975).

There are now a great variety of "buzzer-pad" devices. Lists of manufacturers and their addresses are available for England (Meadow, 1977) and the United States (Mountjoy et al., 1984). Unfortunately in everyday situations, the buzzer-pad device often fails simply because it is not used appropriately (Mountjoy et al., 1984). An instructive article on the use of this procedure has been prepared by Meadow (1977).

An elaboration of the buzzer-pad procedure, called Dry-Bed Training (DBT), was formulated by Azrin et al. (1974). This procedure consists of (a) the buzzer-pad, (b) nighttime awakenings, (c) retention control training, and (d) positive practice and cleanliness training. Briefly, these procedures involve the following: *Nighttime awakening* refers to awakening the child during the night, having the child void in the toilet, and praising him or her for keeping the bed dry. The *retention control training* procedure requires the child to take a large drink of water (at least one pint) before bed. The youngster is then awakened at hourly intervals and asked *not* to urinate unless absolutely necessary. The child is praised for the dry bed and takes another large drink before going to sleep. This is done on the first night only. For *positive practice* the child lies in bed with the lights off, counts silently up to a specified number, and then goes to the bathroom to urinate. The procedure is repeated 20 times. *Cleanliness training* pertains to toiletting accidents. If the child wets the bed (alarm goes off), he or she must change pyjamas and sheets, dry the detector, remake the bed, and perform positive practice. There have been some excellent studies conducted in Australia on various aspects of the DBT procedures (e.g., Bollard, 1982; Bollard & Nettelbeck, 1982), and their findings indicate that DBT is superior to using just the buzzer-pad device. Nevertheless, the buzzer-pad in combination with nighttime awakening is almost equally effective as the whole DBT procedure.

The true effectiveness of enuresis treatment programs is often gauged by the relapse rate (i.e., the percentage of children who begin to wet the bed after the training program has been completed). A reasonable period is 2 years. Unfortunately, about 40% of the children who undergo either DBT or the buzzer-pad procedure experience relapse (e.g., Bollard, 1982). Children who do relapse, however, often achieve bladder control after retraining. Those who have a history of daytime wetting accidents after the age of 4 years are more likely to experience relapses (Bollard, 1982), as are youngsters with behavior problems or who are from stressful family environments (Dische et al., 1983).

Relative Efficacy

The relative efficacy of Tofranil, conditioning, and placebo was investigated in a well-controlled study conducted by Kolvin et al. (1972). Children in the study were separated into three groups, each receiving one of the aforementioned treatments. Therapy for each group lasted 2 months, with the results being evaluated 2 months later. Treatment was considered successful if there was an 80% decrease in wet nights. Using this criterion, 42% of the placebo group, 30% of the medication group, and 50% of the buzzer-pad group were considered improved. Although a number of research questions remain unanswered (Blackwell & Currah, 1972), this study demonstrates the effectiveness of both placebo and conditioning techniques for the management of enuresis as well as the existence of viable alternatives to drug therapy. The debate concerning the relative efficacy of medication versus behavioral interventions will no doubt continue. Another study by Wagner et al. (1982), for example, found tricyclic antidepressants to be superior to the buzzer-pad in a short-term study.

Drug-Induced Enuresis

Drug-induced enuresis is associated primarily with neuroleptic treatment. To date, reports of this side effect in children have been published for Mellaril (thioridazine), Prolixin (fluphenazine), Haldol (haloperidol), and Orap (pimozide) (see Ambrosini, 1984). Children with no history of enuresis may be affected, whereas known enuretics may become "dry" when receiving neuroleptic medication. This side effect appears to be self-limiting.

SEPARATION ANXIETY (SCHOOL PHOBIA)

The distress reaction shown by infants when they are separated from their mothers is referred to as *separation anxiety*. In theory, this reaction is not limited to infants and may be manifest in children and adolescents as school phobia and in adult *agoraphobics* as panic anxiety (Gittelman-Klein, 1975). Agoraphobics "suffer from inexplicable panic attacks, accompanied by hot and cold flashes, rapid breathing, palpitations, weakness, unsteadiness, a feeling of impending death, and occasional depersonalization. They progressively constrict their activities until they are unable to leave the house independently for fear of being suddenly rendered helpless while isolated from help" (Gittelman-Klein & Klein, 1973, p. 200). For obvious reasons this phobia is quite disabling; however, it seems to respond to Tofranil treatment. Interestingly, many adult agoraphobics also suffered from school phobia when they were younger. It was reasoned that drugs (i.e., Tofranil) effective for the control of panic attacks in adult agoraphobics might also be useful for the treatment of school phobia (Gittelman-Klein, 1975). A well-controlled study was conducted to test this hypothesis. Subjects were selected only after intense efforts were made to force the child to return to school. It was found that Tofranil was clearly superior to placebo in enabling school-phobic children to attend school. When effective, medication "frees the child of panicky responses to, and morbid fears during, separation" (Gittelman-Klein, 1975, p. 266).

The average dose of Tofranil for this disorder is 75 to 100 mg per day with a maximum upper limit of 200 mg per day. Although behavioral improvement may be evident immediately after the onset of treatment, it is more characteristically manifested sometime within the first 2 weeks. Medication is often given before bed to avoid side effects (e.g., drowsiness, dry mouth). Total duration of treatment, including a gradual withdrawal period, lasts about 3 months.

Side effects in school-phobic children treated with Tofranil have been found to include dry mouth, nausea, tremors, sweating, dizziness, drowsiness, lethargy, and decreased appetite (Saraf et al., 1974). Also, one death has been reported, a 6-year-old girl who was administered 300 mg (14 mg/kg) of Tofranil before bed for school phobia. It is therefore highly recommended that the daily dose of Tofranil not exceed 5 mg/kg.

To be truly effective, treatment must include psychotherapy as well as the cooperation of the school, family, and child. Behavioral intervention strategies should be attempted before a trial of medication. It should be noted that many children who have a complete remission of symptoms with Tofranil later suffer relapses.

TICS AND TOURETTE SYNDROME

Psychiatrists currently recognize three different types of disorders whose primary or sole clinical features are tics: transient tic of childhood, chronic motor tic, and Tourette syndrome (American Psychiatric Association, 1980). A *tic* is a rapid, rhythmic, involuntary movement (or spasm) of an individual muscle group. Tic disorders are fairly common in children, and it is estimated that 15% of all school-aged youngsters will experience at least one of them at some time during their childhood.

Transient tic of childhood is often characterized by simple motor tics such as eye blinking, nose puckering, grimacing, and squinting. Vocalizations are less common and include such things as throat sounds, sniffing, humming, and other noises. They are called transient because they generally last only a few weeks or a few months. However, a particular child may experience a series of transient tics over the course of several years. They are much more common in males, are generally not associated with behavior disorders or learning disabilities, and are more likely to be exhibited during periods of excitement or stress.

Chronic motor tics occur for many years, and are unchanging (both in terms of symptoms and severity) in nature. Vocal tics are uncommon. Although both of the aforementioned disorders are responsive to drug therapy, they are generally *not* considered to be serious medical problems or treated with medication.

Tourette syndrome has been described in the medical literature for at least 500 years and is named in honor of Gilles de la Tourette for his classic study of the disorder (Gilles de la Tourette, 1885). This can be an extremely debilitating condition and is characterized by multiple, frequently changing motor and vocal (phonic) tics. The diagnosis is based upon the following criteria: (a) an age of onset between 2 and 15 years (mean age = 7 years), (b) multiple involuntary motor and vocal tics, (c) ability to suppress tics voluntarily for minutes to hours, (d) waxing and waning of symptoms (i.e., variations in intensity of symptoms over time), and (e) duration of symptoms for more than 1 year. Motor tics can be separated into two groups, *simple* (fast, darting, and meaningless muscle spasms) and *complex* (slower and more purposeful). Examples of simple motor tics are eye blinking, nose twitching, grimacing, shoulder shrugs, arm or head jerks, finger movements, jaw snaps, and rapid jerking of any body part. Complex motor tics include such things as clapping, throwing, hopping, self-mutilation, touching objects, bending to touch the floor, sticking out the tongue, *echopraxia* (imitating what one has just seen), and so forth. Vocal tics are also varied and include *simple vocal tics* (e.g., whistling, sniffling, barking, grunting, coughing, and so forth), *complex vocal tics* (e.g., saying words, phrases, or statements), *cuprolalia* (saying obscene or aggressive words or statements), *palilalia* (repeating one's own words), and *echolalia* (repeating the words of others). The symptoms of Tourette syndrome can range from mild to severe, show extreme variability in type, frequency and severity over time, and demonstrate situation specificity (*may* be controlled in school but occurs at a distressing level at home, particularly right after school).

In addition to motor and vocal tics, approximately one half of all diagnosed cases of Tourette syndrome also experience the behavioral symptoms of hyperactivity (attention deficits, motor restlessness, poor concentration, and impulsivity; see Comings & Comings, 1984). Learning disabilities and academic underachievement are common, as are obsessions (preoccupation with an idea or desire) and compulsions. Many complain of "inner tension" and an inability to relax like others (Bruun, 1984). The behavioral concomitants of Tourette syndrome may persist into adulthood. The disorder is much more common in males; the IQs of patients are normally distributed; and most children with Tourette syndrome experience satisfactory life adjustment. There is a strong genetic component in

Tourette syndrome, and the offspring of mothers with the disorder are at quite high risk for developing Tourette syndrome.

Tourette syndrome is rare, but there is some controversy regarding its "true" prevalence. Estimates vary but a commonly cited figure is approximately 1 case per 2,000 (or 0.05%) for full-blown Tourette syndrome (Cohen et al., 1984; Shapiro & Shapiro, 1982).

Pharmacotherapy for Tourette Syndrome

At the present time, the only proven effective treatment for the control of motor and vocal tics associated with Tourette syndrome are psychotropic drugs. Several different drugs are currently being used in the pharmacological management of this disorder, each of which is discussed separately. More detailed discussions of pharmacological treatment are available elsewhere (e.g., Cohen et al., 1985; Shapiro & Shapiro, 1981).

Haldol (Haloperidol). Since the 1960s, the drug of first choice for the treatment of Tourette syndrome is Haldol, a neuroleptic (major tranquilizer). Approximately 80% of all people show some initial benefit from medication, but owing primarily to side effects, far less (approximately 20 to 30%) take the drug for extended periods of time. Haldol is very effective at low dosages. The child-patient is generally started on a dose of 0.25 to 0.5 mg per day (administered at bedtime), which is increased every 4 or 5 days (at no more than 0.5 mg increments) to an average daily dose of 3 to 4 mg. Haldol's behavioral half-life is at least 4 days. At low dosages, many patients experience a complete remission of symptoms and few adverse reactions. The more common side effects of Haldol are sedation, excessive fatigue, excessive appetite, weight gain, dysphoria, intellectual dulling, feeling dull or like a zombie, memory problems, and personality changes. The drug may also cause the child to become fearful or school phobic (afraid to go to school) during the first weeks of treatment, which may continue for months if the drug is not discontinued. This reaction abates within weeks of drug withdrawal.

There has, and continues to be, a debate as to whether or not neuroleptic medication impairs academic performance at clinically optimum levels. Unfortunately, few drug researchers actually study classroom learning (Gadow & Swanson, 1985), and there is nothing to suggest that this situation will change. Although there are studies that did find drug-induced cognitive impairment in intellectually normal children treated with Haldol (Platt et al., 1984; Werry

& Aman, 1975) and a mixed group of child and adult Tourette syndrome patients treated with Orap (Shapiro et al., 1984), we are forced to rely on clinical experience with regard to school performance. The following quote from Brunn (1984) summarizing her experience with high dosages of Haldol bears directly on this issue and is particularly relevant in situations in which poor drug monitoring procedures are currently used:

> With such a rapid increase the effective dose level had unknowingly been far exceeded. Although well intentioned, this was a particular disservice to children who could not articulate the changes they were experiencing. True, they were now virtually symptom free. Their parents were usually delighted and tended to overlook some other important ways in which their children had changed. Whereas previously they had been excitable, enthusiastic participants in life, they were now becoming listless, apathetic and withdrawn. They were drifting through school, absorbing just enough to get by. Instead of making the social adjustments of a normal adolescence they were choosing not to participate. They often became clinging and overly dependent on their parents, who tended to be overprotective, possibly to assuage their own guilt for punishments inflicted prior to the diagnosis and for their continuing angry feelings. The high-dose medicated children tended to gain too much weight and to give an overtranquilized appearance which was often mistaken for stupidity. As a result they were avoided by their peers perhaps as much or more than they would have been had they been exhibiting the now suppressed symptoms of TS. (pp. 128–129)

Treatment with Haldol may lead to the appearance of extrapyramidal syndromes such as acute dystonic reactions, akathisia, Parkinsonian syndrome, and tardive dyskinesia. Because these side effects are discussed in Chapter 4, only a few comments are made here. First, parents, the child (when appropriate), and other care providers must be informed of these side effects prior to the onset of treatment. Second, the prophylactic use of anticholinergic drugs (e.g., Cogentin) is not recommended. In other words, an anticholinergic should not be given in combination with Haldol when Haldol is first administered as a way of preventing the appearance of extrapyramidal symptoms. Third, it is important to establish a clear picture of the child's symptoms prior to treatment because extrapyramidal symptoms could be mistaken for tics or the psychological sequellae of the disorder.

Because the symptoms of Tourette syndrome can produce a considerable degree of emotional anguish for a child, the benefits of treatment must be carefully weighed against the risks such as adverse drug reactions and the psychosocial aspects of taking medication. With this said, the following quote from Cohen et al. (1984) is presented:

Side effects of neuroleptics may have considerable impact on a child's sense of self control, autonomy, self esteem, and cognitive and social competence. In addition to the way in which psychoactive medication may alter how a child's body feels to him and how he experiences the working of his mind, the use of any medication may single a child out in school, alter his daily schedule, focus parental and other adult concern on small changes in symptoms and side effects, and tie the child down to the care and attention of many adults. (p. 17)

The withdrawal of Haldol may lead to an exacerbation (worsening) of symptoms to a level far worse than before the onset of medication. This reaction could last for up to 2 to 3 months. Conversely, some children may show improvement following drug discontinuation only to worsen later and gradually improve again. The withdrawal of medication may also be greeted with some relief because side effects such as cognitive blunting dissipate. For these reasons, evaluating the need to continue treatment is a complex process. Not only should the child and caregivers be prepared for these possibilities, but also drug-free periods or dosage reductions should be scheduled to assess the need for medication.

Catapres (Clonidine). The first report of Catapres being an effective agent in the treatment of Tourette syndrome appeared in 1979. In one uncontrolled study, Cohen et al. (1980) reported an improvement rate of 70%. Catapres is approved by the FDA for the treatment of hypertension, but its role in the management of Tourette syndrome is not officially recognized. This situation will probably change, however, when enough studies have been completed. Because children often experience intolerable side effects to Haldol, such as sedation, the search for new agents is important. Catapres appears to be effective for the management of simple and complex motor and vocal tics *and* for improvement of attention deficits. Nevertheless, the findings from more well-controlled studies (e.g., Shapiro et al., 1983) indicate that Catapres is less effective than Haldol and benefits only a small subsample of people with Tourette syndrome. Moreover, there is some discussion that it may be more useful in controlling the associated symptoms such as hyperactivity and inattentiveness.

In the treatment of Tourette syndrome, Catapres is initiated at a small daily dose (0.05 mg) that is gradually increased over several weeks to 0.15 to 0.30 mg per day. Because Catapres has a short half-life (6 hours), it is administered in small doses 3 to 4 times per day. Catapres has a slower onset of action than Haldol and may take 3 weeks or more to produce a therapeutic response. A true evaluation of its efficacy may require waiting for 3 to 4 months after the onset of therapy. Tolerance to beneficial effects is a problem in some children.

The major side effect of Catapres is sedation, but this generally goes away after several weeks. Sedation can have serious consequences. For example, one patient was reportedly involved in a serious auto accident because of this reaction (Shapiro et al., 1983). Teenagers who drive (and their parents) must be warned of the risks associated with drug-induced sedation. This caveat obviously holds for *all* drugs that can produce marked sedation. Other reported side effects include impaired cognition, dry mouth, sensitivity of eyes to light, *bradycardia* (slowness of heart rate), hypotension, dizziness, irritability, nightmares, and insomnia.

Orap (Primozide). Approved by the FDA (United States) in 1984 for the treatment of Tourette syndrome, Orap is a powerful neuroleptic. It is effective for the treatment of Tourette syndrome (e.g., Shapiro & Shapiro, 1984), and uncontrolled studies suggest that it *may* be equally effective as Haldol and less sedating. Treatment is typically initiated with a dosage of 1 mg per day, which is gradually increased to 6 to 10 mg per day (0.2 mg/kg per day). Because Orap has a relatively long half-life (55 hours), it is possible to administer medication once a day. The side effects of Orap are similar to those of Haldol. Because Orap can have an adverse effect on heart function, an EKG should be administered prior to treatment.

Other Drugs. In addition to the drugs already discussed, Tourette syndrome responds to other neuroleptic medication such as Prolixin and penfluridol (not approved for general use in the United States). Some clinicians also report experimentation with multiple-drug therapy, for example, small therapeutic doses of Haldol and Catapres, when side effects or limited efficacy are a problem (see Cohen et al., 1985).

Clinical Considerations

The behavioral concomitants of Tourette syndrome (e.g., hyperactivity), its psychological sequelae (e.g., embarrassment, social rejection, anxiety from not being in control of one's own body), and its associated academic impediments (both drug-induced and preexisting) relegate drug therapy to an adjunctive role in the treatment process. An effort should be made to ensure that the child is receiving an adequate educational program and that his or her emotional needs are being attended to (see Bauer & Shea, 1984).

Given the risks of both behavioral and somatic toxicity, neuro-leptic medication must be carefully monitored. It is very important that parents and other care providers be informed of potential drug effects and be prepared to facilitate their management. Because the child often does not exhibit the full range of symptoms in the physi-cian's office, caregiver reports may be essential in establishing base-line (pretreatment) levels of adaptive and symptomatic behaviors.

It is a well-established fact that stimulant drugs can induce tics and exacerbate the symptoms of Tourette syndrome (Lowe et al., 1982). It is controversial, however, whether or not stimulants can cause this disorder in children who would not otherwise develop it. For this reason, consideration should be given to the prudence of using stimulants for hyperactivity with children who have a first-degree relative (parent, brother, or sister) with Tourette syndrome. Moreover, drug withdrawal should be seriously considered for chil-dren who experience drug-induced tics and who were, prior to treat-ment, tic-free. This too is controversial because tics often abate with dosage reduction.

Lastly, there is a national organization whose efforts are devoted to the welfare of people with Tourette syndrome. Their address is cited here as a source for more information about the disorder and its management.

Tourette Syndrome Association
41–02 Bell Boulevard
Bayside, NY 11361
(718) 224–2999

SUGGESTED READINGS

Azrin, N. H., & Thienes, P. M. (1978). Rapid elimination of enuresis by intensive learning without a conditioning apparatus. *Behavior Therapy, 9,* 342–354. (C, S)

Blackwell, B., & Currah, J. (1972). The psychopharmacology of nocturnal enuresis. In I. Kalvin, R. C. MacKeith, & S. R. Meadow (Eds.), *Bladder control and enuresis* (pp. 231–257). London: Heinemann. (C, S)

Cohen, D. J., Leckman, J. F., & Shaywitz, B. A. (1984). A physician's guide to diagnosis and treatment of Tourette syndrome. Bayside, NY: Tourette Syndrome Association.

Cohen, D. J., Leckman, J. F., & Shaywitz, B. A. (1985). The Tourette syndrome and other tics. In D. Shaffer, A. A. Ehrhardt, & L. L. Greenhill (Eds.), *The clinical guide to child psychiatry* (pp. 3–28). Free Press: New York. (C, S)

Fritz, G. K., & Armbrust, J. (1982). Enuresis and encopresis. *Psychiatric Clinics of North America, 5*, 283–297. (C, S)

Gittelman-Klein, R. (1975). Pharmacotherapy and management of pathological separation anxiety. *International Journal of Mental Health, 4*, 255–271. (C, S)

McLellan, D. L. (1983). The drug treatment of spasticity. *International Rehabilitation Medicine, 5*, 141–142. (C, S)

Mountjoy, P. T., Ruben, D. H., & Bradford, T. S. (1984). Recent technological advancements in the treatment of enuresis. *Behavior Modification, 8*, 291–315. (C, S)

Shapiro, A. K., & Shapiro, E. (1982). An update on Tourette syndrome. *American Journal of Psychotherapy, 36*, 379–390. (C, S)

REFERENCES

Ambrosini, P. J. (1984). A pharmacological paradigm for urinary incontinence and enuresis. *Journal of Clinical Psychopharmacology, 4*, 247–253.

American Psychiatric Association. (1980). *Diagnostic and statistical manual of mental disorders* (3rd ed.). Washington, DC: Author.

Azrin, N. H., Sneed, T. J., & Foxx, R. M. (1974). Dry-Bed: Rapid elimination of childhood enuresis. *Behaviour Research and Therapy, 12*, 147–156.

Azrin, N. H., & Thienes, P. M. (1978). Rapid elimination of enuresis by intensive learning without a conditioning apparatus. *Behavior Therapy, 9*, 342–354.

Baker, H. J. (1959). *Exceptional children* (3rd ed.). New York: Macmillan.

Bauer, A. M., & Shea, T. M. (1984). Tourette syndrome: A review and educational implications. *Journal of Autism and Developmental Disorders, 14*, 69–80.

Blackwell, B., & Currah, J. (1972). The psychopharmacology of nocturnal enuresis. In I. Kalvin, R. C. MacKeith, & S. R. Meadow (Eds.), *Bladder control and enuresis* (pp. 231–257). London: Heinemann.

Bollard, J. (1982). A 2-year follow-up of bedwetters treated by dry-bed training and standard conditioning. *Behaviour Research and Therapy, 20*, 571–580.

Bollard, J., & Nettelbeck, T. (1982). A component analysis of Dry-Bed Training for treatment for bedwetting. *Behaviour Research and Therapy, 20*, 383–390.

Bruun, R. D. (1984). Gilles de la Tourette's syndrome: An overview of clinical experience. *Journal of the American Academy of Child Psychiatry, 23*, 126–133.

Cohen, D. J., Detlor, J., Young, J. G., & Shaywitz, B. A. (1980). Clonidine ameliorates Gilles de la Tourette syndrome. *Archives of General Psychiatry, 37*, 1350–1357.

Cohen, D. J., Leckman, J. F., & Shaywitz, B. A. (1984). The Tourette syndrome and other tics. In D. Shaffer, A. A. Ehrhardt, & L. L. Greenhill (Eds.), *The clinical guide to child psychiatry* (pp. 3–28). Free Press: New York.

Comings, D. E., & Comings, B. G. (1984). Tourette's syndrome and attention deficit disorder with hyperactivity: Are they genetically related? *Journal of the American Academy of Child Psychiatry, 23,* 138–146.

Cronin, A. J., Khalil, R., & Little, T. M. (1979). Poisoning with tricyclic antidepressants: An avoidable cause of childhood deaths. *British Medical Journal, 1,* 722.

Cruickshank, W. M., & Raus, G. M. (1955). Size and scope of the problem. In W. M. Cruickshank & G. M. Raus (Eds.), *Cerebral palsy: Its individual and community problems* (2nd ed., pp. 1–20). Syracuse: Syracuse University Press.

Denhoff, E., Feldman, S., Smith, M. G., Litchman, H., & Holden, W. (1975). Treatment of spastic cerebral-palsied children with sodium dantrolene. *Developmental Medicine and Child Neurology, 17,* 736–742.

Diamond, J. M., & Stein, J. M. (1983). Enuresis: A new look at stimulant therapy. *Canadian Journal of Psychiatry, 28,* 395–397.

Dische, S., Yule, W., Corbett, J., & Hand, D. (1983). Childhood nocturnal enuresis: Factors associated with outcome of treatment with an enuresis alarm. *Developmental Medicine and Child Neurology, 25,* 67–80.

Domino, E. F. (1974). Centrally acting skeletal-muscle relaxants. *Archives of Physical Medicine and Rehabilitation, 55,* 369–373.

Dunsdon, M. I. (1952). *The educability of cerebral palsied children.* London: Newnes Educational.

Forsythe, W. I., & Redmond, A. (1974). Enuresis and spontaneous cure rate. *Archives of Disease in Childhood, 49,* 259–263.

Gadow, K. D., & Swanson, H. L. (1985). Assessing drug effects on academic performance. *Psychopharmacology Bulletin, 21,* 877–885. *Journal of Mental Deficiency, 85,* 588–595.

Gadow, K. D., & Swanson, H. L. (in press). Assessing drug effects on academic performance. *Psychopharmacology Bulletin.*

Gilles de la Tourette, G. (1885). Etude sur une affection nerveuse caraterisee par de l'incoordination motrice accompagnée d'echolalie et de copralalie. *Archives de Neurologie, 9,* 19–42, 158–200.

Gittelman-Klein, R. (1975). Pharmacotherapy and management of pathological separation anxiety. *International Journal of Mental Health, 4,* 255–271.

Gittelman-Klein, R., & Klein, D. F. (1973). School phobia: Diagnostic considerations in the light of imipramine effects. *Journal of Nervous and Mental Disease, 156,* 199–215.

Kendall, P. H. (1964). The use of muscle relaxants in cerebral palsy. In E. Denhoff (Ed.), *Drugs in cerebral palsy* (Clinics in Developmental Medicine No. 16). London: Heinemann.

Kolvin, I., Taunch, J., Currah, J., Garside, R. F., Nolan, J., & Shaw, W. B. (1972). Enuresis—a descriptive analysis and a controlled trial. *Developmental Medicine and Child Neurology, 14,* 715–726.

Lowe, T. L., Cohen, D. J., Detlor, J., Kremenitzer, M. W., & Shaywitz, B. A. (1982). Stimulant medications precipitate Tourette's syndrome. *Journal of the American Medical Association, 247,* 1729–1731.

MacLean, R. E. G. (1960). Imipramine hydrochloride and enuresis. *American Journal of Psychiatry, 117,* 551.

McLellan, D. L. (1983). The drug treatment of spasticity. *International Rehabilitation Medicine, 5,* 141–142.

Meadow, R. (1977). How to use buzzer alarms to cure bed-wetting. *British Medical Journal, 2,* 1073–1075.

Meadow, R., & Berg, I. (1982). Controlled trial of imipramine in diurnal enuresis. *Archives of Disease in Childhood, 57,* 714–716.

Molitch, M., & Poliakoff, S. (1937). Effects of benzedrine sulfate on enuresis. *Archives of Pediatrics, 54,* 499–501.

Mountjoy, P. T., Ruben, D. H., & Bradford, T. S. (1984). Recent technological advancements in the treatment of enuresis. *Behavior Modification, 8,* 291–315.

Mowrer, O. H. (1938). Apparatuses for the study and treatment of enuresis. *American Journal of Psychology, 51,* 163–165.

Mowrer, O. H. (1950). *Learning theory and personality dynamics.* New York: Ronald Press.

Parkin, J. M., & Fraser, M. S. (1972). Poisoning as a complication of enuresis. *Developmental Medicine and Child Neurology, 14,* 727–730.

Perlstein, M. A. (1955). Infantile cerebral palsy. *Advances in Pediatrics, 7,* 209–248.

Platt, J. E., Campbell, M., Green, W. H., & Grega, D. M. (1984). Cognitive effects of lithium carbonate and haloperidol in treatment-resistant aggressive children. *Archives of General Psychiatry, 120,* 657–662.

Roberts, M. H. W., & Wright, V. (1983). Drugs or physical therapy in rehabilitation. *International Rehabilitation Medicine, 5,* 29–31.

Robison, D. S., & Barker, E. (1976). Tricyclic antidepressant cardiotoxicity. *Journal of the American Medical Association, 236,* 2089–2090.

Saraf, K. R., Klein, D. F., Gittelman-Klein, R., & Groff, S. (1974). Imipramine side effects in children. *Psychopharmacologia, 37,* 265–274.

Shapiro, A. K., & Shapiro, E. (1981). The treatment and etiology of tics and Tourette syndrome. *Comprehensive Psychiatry, 22,* 193–205.

Shapiro, A. K., & Shapiro, E. (1982). An update on Tourette syndrome. *American Journal of Psychotherapy, 36,* 379–390.

Shapiro, A. K., & Shapiro, E. (1984). Controlled study of pimozide vs. placebo in Tourette's syndrome. *Journal of the American Academy of Child Psychiatry, 2,* 161–173.

Shapiro, A. K., Shapiro, E., & Eisenkraft, G. J. (1983). Treatment of Gilles de la Tourette's syndrome with clonidine and neuroleptics. *Archives of General Psychiatry, 40,* 1235–1240.

Shapiro, E., Shapiro, A. K., & Levine, R. (1984, October). *The effect of pimozide on cognition.* Paper presented at the meeting of the American Academy of Child Psychiatry, Toronto.

Stewart, M. A. (1975). Treatment of bedwetting. *Journal of the American Medical Association, 232,* 281–283.

Wagner, W., Johnson, S. B., Walker, D., Carter, R., & Wittner, J. (1982). A controlled comparison of two treatments for nocturnal enuresis. *Journal of Pediatrics, 101,* 302–307.

Werry, J. S. (1965). Emotional factors and enuresis nocturna. *Developmental Medicine and Child Neurology, 7,* 563–565.

Werry, J. S., & Aman, M. G. (1975). Methylphenidate and haloperidol in children. *Archives of General Psychiatry, 32,* 790–795.

APPENDIX A

Classification of Selected Psychotropic Drugs

Generic Name	Trade Name*

1. Stimulants

Amphetamine	Benzedrine
Deanol	Deaner
Dextroamphetamine	Dexedrine
Methamphetamine	Desoxyn
Methylphenidate	Ritalin
Pemoline	Cylert

2. Antidepressants

Tricyclics

Amitriptyline	Elavil, Endep
Desipramine	Norpramin, Pertofrane
Doxepin	Adapin, Sinequan
Imipramine	Janimine, SK-Pramine, Tofranil
Nortriptyline	Aventyl, Pamelor
Protriptyline	Vivactil
Trimipramine	Surmontil

Monoamine Oxidase Inhibitors

Isocarboxazid	Marplan
Phenelzine	Nardil
Tranylcypromine	Parnate

Appendix A (Continued)

Generic Name	Trade Name*

3. Antianxiety Agents (Minor Tranquilizers)

Propanediols

Meprobamate	Equanil, Miltown

Diphenylmethane

Hydroxyzine	Atarax, Durrax, Vistaril

Benzodiazepines

Alprazolam	Xanax
Chlordiazepoxide	Librium
Clonazepam	Clonopin
Clorazepate	Tranxene
Diazepam	Valium
Flurazepam	Dalmane
Halazepam	Paxipam
Lorazepam	Ativan
Oxazepam	Serax
Prazepam	Centrax
Temazepam	Restoril
Triazolam	Halcion

4. Neuroleptics (Antipsychotics, Major Tranquilizers)

Phenothiazines

a. Aliphatic

Chlorpromazine	Thorazine
Promazine	Sparine
Triflupromazine	Vesprin

b. Piperdine

Piperacetazine	Quide
Mesoridazine	Serentil
Thioridazine	Mellaril

c. Piperazine

Acetophenazine	Tindal
Fluphenazine	Prolixin, Permitil
Perphenazine	Trilafon
Prochlorperazine	Compazine
Trifluoperazine	Stelazine

Thioxanthenes

Chlorprothixene	Taractan
Thiothixene	Navane

Butyrophenone

Haloperidol	Haldol

Appendix A (Continued)

Generic Name	Trade Name*
	Dihydroindolone
Molindone	Moban
	Dibenzoxazepine
Amoxapine	Asendin
Loxapine	Loxitane
	Diphenylbutylpiperidine
Pimozide	Orap

5. Sedative—Hypnotics

	Barbiturates
Amobarbital	Amytal
Aprobarbital	Alurate
Butabarbital	Butisol
Mephobarbital	Mebaral
Pentobarbital	Nembutal
Phenobarbital	Luminal
Secobarbital	Seconal
	Nonbarbiturates
Chloral hydrate	Noctec
Ethchlorvynol	Placidyl
Ethinamate	Valmid
Glutethimide	Doriden
Methaqualone	Quaalude, Sopor
Methyprylon	Noludar

6. Anticholinergic Drugs

Benztropine	Cogentin
Biperiden	Akineton
Ethopropazine	Parsidol
Trihexyphenidyl	Artane
Procyclidine	Kemadrin

7. Other Therapeutic Agents

Lithium carbonate	Eskalith, Lithane
	Lithonate

*Only trade name products marketed in the United States are listed. In the case of drugs no longer protected by patent laws, the inclusion of trade names other than the original was arbitrary.

APPENDIX B

Classification of the Epilepsies

I. PARTIAL (FOCAL, LOCAL) SEIZURES

Partial seizures are those in which, in general, the first clinical and electroencephalographic changes indicate initial activation of a system of neurons limited to part of one cerebral hemisphere. A partial seizure is classified primarily on the basis of whether or not consciousness is impaired during the attack. When consciousness is not impaired, tho sei zure is classifiod as a simple partial seizure. When consciousness is impaired, the seizure is classified as a complex partial seizure. Impairment of consciousness may be the first clinical sign, or simple partial seizures may evolve into complex partial seizures. In patients with impaired consciousness, aberrations of behavior (automatisms) may occur. A partial seizure may not terminate but instead may progress to a generalized motor seizure. Impaired consciousness is defined as the inability to respond normally to exogenous stimuli by virtue of altered awareness and/or responsiveness (see following section, Definition of Terms).

There is considerable evidence that simple partial seizures usually have unilateral hemispheric involvement and only rarely have bilateral hemispheric involvement; complex partial seizures, however, frequently have bilateral hemispheric involvement.

Partial seizures can be classified into one of the following three fundamental groups: a) simple partial seizures; b) complex partial seizures; c) partial seizures evolving to generalized tonic-clonic convulsions (GTC).

A. Simple Partial Seizures

CLINICAL SEIZURE TYPE: Simple partial seizures: consciousness not impaired.

EEG SEIZURE TYPE: Local contralateral discharge starting over the corresponding area of cortical representation (not always recorded on the scalp).

EEG INTERICTAL EXPRESSION: Local contralateral discharge.

1. With motor signs
   a. focal motor without march
   b. focal motor with march (Jacksonian)
   c. versive
   d. postural
   e. phonatory (vocalization or arrest of speech)

2. With autonomic symptoms (including epigastric sensation, pallor, sweating, flushing, piloerection, and pupillary dilatation)

3. With somatosensory or special sensory symptoms (simple hallucinations, e.g., tingling, light flashes, buzzing)

   a. somatosensory
   b. visual
   c. auditory
   d. olfactory
   e. gustatory
   f. vertiginous

4. With psychic symptoms (disturbance of higher cerebral function). These rarely occur without impairment of consciousness and are more commonly seen as complex partial seizures.

   a. dysphasic
   b. dysmnesic (e.g., déjà vu)
   c. cognitive (e.g., dreamy states, distortions of time sense)
   d. affective (fear, anger, and other emotional states)
   e. illusions (e.g., macropsia)
   f. structured hallucinations (e.g., music, scenes)

B. Complex Partial Seizures

CLINICAL SEIZURE TYPE: Complex partial seizure: with impairment of consciousness; may sometimes begin with simple symptomatology.

EEG SEIZURE TYPE: Unilateral or, frequently, bilateral discharge, diffuse or focal in temporal or frontotemporal regions.

EEG INTERICTAL EXPRESSION: Unilateral or bilateral, generally asynchronous focus; usually in the temporal regions.

1. Simple partial onset followed by impairment of consciousness
   a. with simple partial features (A1–A4) followed by impaired consciousness
   b. with automatisms

2. With impairment of consciousness at onset
   a. with impairment of consciousness only
   b. with automatisms

C. Partial Seizures Evolving to Generalized Tonic-Clonic Seizures (GTC)

CLINICAL SEIZURE TYPE: GTC with partial or focal onset
EEG SEIZURE TYPE: Discharges like those for complex partial seizures, becoming secondarily and rapidly generalized.

1. Simple partial seizures (A) evolving to GTC

2. Complex partial (B) evolving to GTC

3. Simple partial seizures evolving to complex partial seizures evolving to GTC

II. GENERALIZED SEIZURES (CONVULSIVE OR NONCONVULSIVE)

Generalized seizures are those in which the first clinical changes indicate initial involvement of both hemispheres. Consciousness may be impaired and this impairment may be the initial manifestation. Motor manifestations are bilateral. The ictal electroencephalographic patterns initially are bilateral and presumably reflect neuronal discharge that is widespread in both hemispheres.

A. Absence Seizures
1. Typical absence siezures (b-f may be used alone or in combination)
   a. impairment of consciousness only
   b. with mild clonic components
   c. with atonic components
   d. with tonic components
   e. with automatisms
   f. with autonomic components

CLINICAL SEIZURE TYPE: Absence seizure.
EEG SEIZURE TYPE: Usually regular and symmetrical 3-Hz activity, but may be 2- to 4-Hz spike-and-slow-wave complexes and may have multiple spike-and-slow-wave complexes. Abnormalities are bilateral.
EEG INTERICTAL EXPRESSION: Background activity is usually normal, although paroxysmal activity (such as spikes or spike-and-slow-wave complexes) may occur.
This activity is usually regular and symmetrical.

2. Atypical absence seizures: may have
   a. changes in tone that are more pronounced
   b. onset and/or cessation that is not abrupt

EEG SEIZURE TYPE: More heterogeneous; may include irregular spike-and-slow-wave complexes, fast activity, or other paroxysmal activity. Abnormalities are bilateral but often irregular and asymmetrical.
EEG INTERICTAL EXPRESSION: Background usually abnormal; a paroxysmal activity (such as spikes or spike-and-slow-wave complexes) frequently irregular and asymmetrical.

B. Tonic-Clonic Seizures

EEG SEIZURE TYPE: Rhythm at 10 or more cycles per second, decreasing in frequency and increasing in amplitude during tonic phase, interrupted by slow waves during clonic phase.
EEG INTERICTAL EXPRESSION: Polyspike-and-wave discharges, spike-and-wave discharges, or sometimes sharp-and-slow-wave discharges.

C. Myoclonic Seizures

CLINICAL SEIZURE TYPE: Myoclonic jerks (single or multiple).
EEG SEIZURE TYPE: Polyspike-and-wave discharges, or sometimes spike-and-wave or sharp-and-slow-wave discharges.
EEG INTERICTAL EXPRESSION: Same pattern as in ictal period

D. Clonic Seizures

EEG SEIZURE TYPE: Fast activity (10 cycles per second or more) and slow waves; occasional spike-and-slow-wave patterns.
EEG INTERICTAL EXPRESSION: Spike-and-wave or polyspike-and-wave discharges.

E. Tonic Seizures

EEG SEIZURE TYPE: Low-voltage, fast activity or a fast rhythm (9-10 cycles per second or more) decreasing in frequency and increasing in amplitude.
EEG INTERICTAL EXPRESSION: More or less rhythmic discharges of sharp and slow waves, sometimes symmetrical.

F. Atonic Seizures

EEG SEIZURE TYPE: Polyspikes and wave discharges or flattening or low-voltage fast activity.
EEG INTERICTAL EXPRESSION: Polyspikes and wave activity.

III. UNCLASSIFIED EPILEPTIC SEIZURES

Includes all seizures that cannot be classified because of inadequate or incomplete data and some that defy classification in hitherto described categories. This includes some neonatal seizures, e.g., rhythmic eye movements, chewing, and swimming movements.

ADDENDUM

1. Repeated epileptic seizures occur under a variety of circumstances:
    a. as fortuitous attacks, coming unexpectedly and without any apparent provocation
    b. as cyclic attacks, at more or less regular intervals (e.g., in relation to the menstrual cycle or to the sleep-waking cycle)
    c. as attacks provoked by 1) nonsensory factors (fatigue, alcohol, emotion) or 2) sensory factors, and sometimes referred to as "reflex seizures"
2. Prolonged or repetitive seizures (status epilepticus). The term "status epilepticus" is used whenever a seizure persists for a sufficient length of time or is repeated frequently enough that recovery between attacks does not occur. Status epilepticus may be devided into partial (e.g., Jacksonian) or generalized (e.g., absence status or tonic-clonic status). When very localized motor status occurs, it is referred to as epilepsia partialis continua.

DEFINITION OF TERMS

Each seizure type will be described so that the criteria used will not be in doubt.

Partial Seizures

The fundamental distinction between simple partial seizures and complex partial seizures is the presence or the impairment of the fully conscious state.

Consciousness has been defined as "that integrating activity by which Man grasps the totality of his phenomenal field" (Evans, 1972) and incorporates it into his experience. It corresponds to "Bewusstsein" and is thus much more than "Vigilance," for were it only vigilance (which is a degree of clarity) then only confusional states would be representative of disordered consciousness.

Operationally in the contest of this classification, *consciousness* refers to the degree of awareness and/or responsiveness of the patient to externally applied stimuli. *Responsiveness* refers to the ability of the patient to carry out simple commands or willed movement and *awareness* refers to the patient's contact with events during the period in question and its recall. A person aware and unresponsive will be able to recount the events that occurred during an attack and his inability to respond by movement or speech. In this context, unresponsiveness is other than the result of paralysis, aphasia or apraxia.

A. *Partial Seizures*

1. With *motor signs.* Any portion of the body may be involved in focal seizure activity depending on the site of origin of the attack in the motor strip. Focal motor seizures may remain strictly focal or they may spread to contiguous cortical areas producing a sequential involvement of body parts in an epileptic "march." The seizure is then known as a Jacksonian seizure. Consciousness is usually preserved; however, the discharge may spread to those structures whose participation is likely to result in loss of consciousness and generalized convulsive movements. Other focal motor attacks may be versive with head turning to one side, usually contraversive to the discharge. If speech is involved, this is either in the form of speech arrest or occasionally vocalization. Occasionally a partial dysphasia is seen in the form of epileptic pallilalia with involuntary repetition of a syllable or phrase.

Following focal seizure activity, there may be a localized paralysis in the previously involved region. This is known as Todd's paralysis and may last from minutes to hours.

When focal motor seizure activity is continuous it is known as epilepsia partialis continua.

2. *Seizures with autonomic symptoms* such as vomiting, pallor, flushing, sweating, piloerection, pupil dilatation, broborygmi, and incontinence may occur as simple partial seizures.

3. *With somatosensory or special sensory symptoms.* Somatosensory seizures as in A.1. Special sensory seizures include visual seizures vary-they are usually described as pins-and-needles or a feeling of numbness. Occasionally a disorder of proprioception or spatial perception occurs. Like motor seizures, somatosensory seizures also may march and also may spread at any time to become complex partial or generalized tonic-clonic seizures as in A.1. Special sensory seizures include visual seizures vary-ing in elaborateness and depending on whether the primary or association areas are involved, from flashing lights to structured visual hallucinatory phenomena, including persons, scenes, etc. (see A.4.f.). Like visual sei-zures, auditory seizures may also run the gamut from crude auditory sensa-tions to such highly integrated functions as music (see A.4.f.). Olfactory sensations, usually in the form of unpleasant odors, may occur.

Gustatory sensations may be pleasant or odious taste hallucinations. They vary in elaboration from crude (salty, sour, sweet, bitter) to sophisti-cated. They are frequently described as "metallic."

Vertiginous symptoms include sensations of falling in space, floating, as well as rotatory vertigo in a horizontal or vertical plane.

4. *With psychic symptoms* (disturbance of higher cerebral function). These usually occur with impairment of consciousness (i.e., complex par-tial seizures).

a. Dysphasia. This was referred to earlier.
b. Dysmnesic symptoms. A distorted memory experience such as distortion of the time sense, a dreamy state, a flashback, or a sensation as if a naive experience had been experienced before, known as déjà vu, or as if a previously experienced sensation had not been experienced, known as jamais-vu, may occur. When this refers to auditory experiences these are known as déjà-entendu or jamais-entendu. Occasionally as a form of forced thinking, the patient may experience a rapid recollection of epi-sodes from his past life, known as panoramic vision.
c. Cognitive disturbances may be experienced. These include dreamy states; distortions of the time sense; sensations of unreality, detachment, or depersonalization.
d. With affective symptomatology. Sensation of extreme pleasure or dis-pleasure, as well as fear and intense depression with feelings of unwor-thiness and rejection may be experienced during seizures. Unlike those of psychiatrically induced depression, these symptoms tend to come in attacks lasting for a few minutes. Anger or rage is occasionally experi-enced, but unlike temper tantrums, epileptic anger is apparently unpro-voked and abates rapidly. Fear or terror is the most frequent symptom; it is sudden in onset, usually unprovoked, and may lead to running away. Associated with the terror, there are frequently objective signs of auto-nomic activity, including pupil dilatation, pallor, flushing, piloerection, palpitation, and hypertension.

   Epileptic or gelastic seizure laughter should not, strictly speaking, be classed as an affective symptom because the laughter is usually with-out affect and hollow. Like other forms of pathological laughter it is often unassociated with true mirth.
e. Illusions. These take the form of distorted perceptions in which objects may appear deformed. Polyoptic illusions such as monocular diplopia,

distortions of size (macropsia or micropsia) or of distance may occur. Similarly, distortions of sound, including microacusia and macroacusia, may be experienced. Depersonalization, as if the person were outside his body, may occur. Altered perception of size or weight of a limb may be noted.

f. Structured hallucinations. Hallucinations may occur as manifestations or perceptions without a corresponding external stimulus and may affect somatosensory, visual, auditory, olfactory, or gustatory senses. If the seizure arises from the primary receptive area, the hallucination would tend to be rather primitive. In the case of vision, flashing lights may be seen; in the case of auditory perception, rushing noises may occur. With more elaborate seizures involving visual or auditory association areas with participation of mobilized memory traces, formed hallucinations occur and these may take the form of scenery, persons, spoken sentences, or music. The character of these perceptions may be normal or distorted.

B.   Seizures with Complex Symptomatology

Automatisms. (These may occur in both partial and generalized seizures. They are described in detail here for convenience.) In the *Dictionary of Epilepsy* (Gastaut, 1973), automatisms are described as "more or less coordinated adapted (eupractic or dyspractic) involuntary motor activity occurring during the state of clouding of consciousness either in the course of, or after an epileptic seizure, and usually followed by amnesia for the event. The automatism may be simply a continuation of an activity that was going on when the seizure occurred, or, conversely, a new activity developed in association with the ictal impairment of consciousness. Usually, the activity is commonplace in nature, often provoked by the subject's environment, or by his sensations during the seizure; exceptionally, fragmentary, primitive, infantile, or antisocial behavior is seen. From a symptomatological point of view the following are distinguished: a) eating automatisms (chewing, swallowing); b) automatisms of mimicry, expressing the subject's emotional state (usually of fear) during the seizure; c) gestural automatisms, crude or elaborate; directed toward either the subject or his environment; d) ambulatory automatisms; e) verbal automatisms."

Ictal epileptic automatisms usually represent the release of automatic behavior under the influence of clouding of consciousness that accompanies a generalized or partial epileptic seizure (confusional automatisms). They may occur in complex partial seizures as well as in absence seizures. Postictal epileptic automatisms may follow any severe epileptic seizure, especially a tonic-clonic one, and are usually associated with confusion.

While some regard masticatory or oropharyngeal automatisms as arising from the amygdala or insular and opercular regions, these movements are occasionally seen in the generalized epilepsies, particularly absence seizures, and are not of localizing help. The same is true of mimicry and gestural automatisms. In the latter, fumbling of the clothes, scratching, and other complex motor activity may occur both in complex partial and absence seizures. Ictal speech automatisms are occasionally encountered. Ambulatory seizures again may occur either as prolonged automatisms of absence, particularly prolonged absence continuing, or of complex partial seizures. In the latter, a patient may occasionally continue to drive a car, although may contravene traffic light regulations.

There seems to be little doubt that automatisms are a common feature of different types of epilepsy. While they do not lend themselves to simple anatomic interpretation, they appear to have in common a discharge involving various areas of the limbic system. Crude and elaborate automatisms do occur in patients with absence as well as complex partial seizures. Of greater significance is the precise descriptive history of the seizures, the age of the patient, the presence or absence of an aura and of postictal behavior including the presence or absence of confusion. The EEG is of cardinal localizational importance here.

Drowsiness or somnolence implies a sleep state from which the patient can be aroused to make appropriate motor and verbal responses. In stupor, the patient may make some spontaneous movement and can be aroused by painful or other vigorously applied stimuli to make avoidance movements. The patient in confusion makes inappropriate responses to his environment and is disoriented as regards place or time or person.

Aura.   A frequently used term in the description of epileptic seizures is aura. According to the *Dictionary of Epilepsy,* this term was introduced by Galen to describe the sensation of a breath of air felt by some subjects prior to the onset of a seizure. Others have referred to the aura as the portion of a seizure experienced before loss of consciousness occurs. This loss of consciousness may be the result of secondary generalization of the seizure discharge or of alteration of consciousness imparted by the development of a complex partial seizure.

The aura is that portion of the seizure which occurs before consciousness is lost and for which memory is retained afterwards. It may be that, as in simple partial seizures, the aura is the whole seizure. Where consciousness is subsequently lost, the aura is, in fact, the signal symptom of a complex partial seizure.

An aura is a retrospective term which is described after the seizure is ended.

Generalized Seizures

A.   Absence Seizures

The hallmark of the absence attack is a sudden onset, interruption of ongoing activities, a blank stare, possibly a brief upward rotation of the eyes. If the patient is speaking, speech is slowed or interrupted: if walking, he stands transfixed; if eating, the food will stop on his way to the mouth. Usually the patient will be unresponsive when spoken to. In some, attacks are aborted when the patient is spoken to. The attack lasts from a few seconds to half a minute and evaporates as rapidly as it commenced.

1. *Absence with impairment of consciousness only.*   The above description fits the description of absence simple in which no other activities take place during the attack.

2. *Absence with mild clonic components.*   Here the onset of the attack is indistinguishable from the above, but clonic movements may occur in the eyelids, at the corner of the mouth, or in other muscle groups which may vary in severity from almost imperceptible movements to generalized myoclonic jerks. Objects held in the hand may be dropped.

3. *Absence with atonic components.*   Here there may be a diminution in tone of muscles subserving posture as well as in the limbs leading to drooping of the head, occasionally slumping of the trunk, dropping of the arms, and relaxation of the grip. Rarely, tone is sufficiently diminished to cause this person to fall.

4. *Absence with tonic components.*   Here during the attack tonic muscular contractions may occur, leading to increase in muscle tone which may affect the extensor muscles or the flexor muscles symmetrically or asymmetrically. If the patient is standing the head may be drawn backward and the trunk may arch. This may lead to retropulsion. The head may tonically draw to one or another side.

5. *Absence with automatisms.*   (See also prior discussion on automatisms.) Purposeful or quasipurposeful movements occurring in the absence of awareness during an absence attack are frequent and may range from lip licking and swallowing to clothes fumbling or aimless walking. If spoken to the patient may grunt or turn to the spoken voice and when touched or tickled may rub the site. Automatisms are quite elaborate and may consist of combinations of the above-described movements or may be so simple as to be missed by casual observation. Mixed forms of absence frequently occur.

B.   Tonic-Clonic Seizures

The most frequently encountered of the generalized seizures are the generalized tonic-clonic seizures, often known as grand mal. Some patients experience a vague ill-described warning, but the majority lose consciousness without any premonitory symptoms. There is a sudden sharp tonic contraction of muscles, and when this involves the respiratory muscles there is stridor, a cry or moan, and the patient falls to the ground in the tonic state, occasionally injuring himself in falling. He lies rigid, and during this stage tonic contraction inhibits respiration and cyanosis may occur. The tongue may be bitten and urine may be passed involuntarily. This tonic stage then gives way to clonic convulsive movements lasting for a variable period of time. During this stage small gusts of grunting respiration may occur between the convulsive movements, but usually the patient remains cyanotic and saliva may froth from the mouth. At the end of this stage, deep respiration occurs and all the muscles relax, after which the patient remains unconscious for a variable period of time and often awakes feeling stiff and sore all over. He then frequently goes into a deep sleep and when he awakens feels quite well apart from soreness and frequently headache. Generalized tonic-clonic convulsions may occur in childhood and in adult life; they are not as frequent as absence seizures, but vary from one a day to one every three months and occasionally to one every few years.

Very short attacks without postictal drowsiness may occur on occasion.

Myoclonic Seizures

Myoclonic jerks (single or multiple) are sudden, brief, shock-like contractions which may be generalized or confined to the face and trunk or to one or more extremities or even to individual muscles or groups of muscles.

Myoclonic jerks may be rapidly repetitive or relatively isolated. They may occur predominantly around the hours of going to sleep or awakening from sleep. They may be exacerbated by volitional movement (action myoclonus). At times they may be regularly repetitive.

Many instances of myoclonic jerks and action myoclonus are not classified as epileptic seizures. The myoclonic jerks of myoclonus due to spinal cord disease, dyssynergia cerebellaris myoclonica, subcortical segmental myoclonus, paramyoclonus multiplex, and opsoclonus-myoclonus syndrome must be distinguished from epileptic seizures.

Clonic Seizures

Generalized convulsive seizures occasionally lack a tonic component and are characterized by repetitive clonic jerks. As the frequency diminishes the amplitude of the jerks do not. The postictal phase is usually short. Some generalized convulsive seizures commence with a clonic phase passing into a tonic phase, as described below, leading to a "clonic-tonic-clonic" seizure.

Tonic Seizures

To quote Gowers, a tonic seizure is "a rigid, violent muscular contraction, fixing the limbs in some strained position. There is usually deviation of the eyes and of the head toward one side, and this may amount to rotation involving the whole body (sometimes actually causing the patient to turn around, even two or three times). The features are distorted; the color of the face, unchanged at first, rapidly becomes pale and then flushed and ultimately livid as the fixation of the chest by the spasms stops the movements of respiration. The eyes are open or closed; the conjunctiva is insensitive; the pupils dilate widely as cyanosis comes on. As the spasm continues, it commonly changes in its relative intensity in different parts, causing slight alterations in the position of the limbs."

Tonic axial seizures with extension of head, neck, and trunk may also occur.

Atonic Seizures

A sudden diminution in muscle tone occurs which may be fragmentary, leading to a head drop with slackening of the jaw, the dropping of a limb or a loss of all muscle tone leading to a slumping to the ground. When these attacks are extremely brief they are known as "drop attacks." If consciousness is lost, this loss is extremely brief. The sudden loss of postural tone in the head and trunk may lead to injury by projecting objects. The face is particularly subject to injury. In the case of more prolonged atonic attacks, the slumping may be progressive in a rhythmic, successive relaxation manner.

(So-called drop attacks may be seen in conditions other than epilepsy, such as brainstem ischemia and narcolepsy cataplexy syndrome.)

Unclassified Epileptic Seizures

This category includes all seizures that cannot be classified because of inadequate or incomplete data and includes some seizures that by their natures defy classification in the previously defined broad categories. Many seizures occurring in the infant (e.g., rhythmic eye movements, chewing, swimming movements, jittering, and apnea) will be classified here until such time as further experience with video-tape confirmation and electroencephalographic characterization entitles them to subtyping in the extant classification.

Epilepsia Partialis Continua

Under this name have been described cases of simple partial seizures with focal motor signs without a march, usually consisting of clonic spasms, which remain confined to the part of the body in which they originate, but which persists with little or no intermission for hours or days at a stretch. Consciousness is usually preserved, but postictal weakness is frequently evident.

Postictal Paralysis (Todd's Paralysis)

This category refers to the transient paralysis that may occur following some partial epileptic seizures with focal motor components or with somatosensory symptoms. Postictal paralysis has been ascribed to neuronal exhaustion due to the increased metabolic activity of the discharging focus, but it may also be attributable to increased inhibition in the region of the focus, which may account for its appearance in nonmotor somatosensory seizures.

REFERENCES

Evans P. Henri Ey's concept of the organization of consciousness and its disorganization: An extension of Jacksonian theory. *Brain* 95:413–440, 1970.

Gastaut H. Clinical and electroencephalographic classification of epileptic seizures. *Epilepsia* 11:102, 1970.

Gastaut H. Definitions. In: *Dictionary of Epilepsy*, Part 1. World Health Organization, Geneva, 1973.

Jackson, J. H. In: Taylor J. A. (Ed.), *Selected Writing of J. Hughlings Jackson, Vol. 1: On Epilepsy and Epileptiform Convulsions*. Hodder and Staughton, London, 1931.

APPENDIX C

Alphabetical List of Selected Psychotropic and Antiepileptic Drugs by Generic Name With Corresponding Trade Name (United States) and Drug Classification

Generic Name	Trade Name*	Classification
Acetazolamide	Diamox	Antiepileptic, Diuretic
Acetophenazine	Tindal	Antipsychotic
Alprazolam	Xanax	Antianxiety
Amantadine	Symmetrel	Antiparkinsonism
Amitriptyline	Elavil, Endep	Antidepressant
Amobarbital	Amytal	Sedative, Hypnotic
Amoxapine	Asendin	Antidepressant
Amphetamine	Benzedrine	Stimulant
Aprobarbital	Alurate	Sedative, Hypnotic
Benztropine	Cogentin	Anticholinergic, Antiparkinsonism
Biperiden	Akineton	Anticholinergic, Antiparkinsonism
Butabarbital	Butisol	Sedative, Hypnotic
Carbamazepine	Tegretol	Antiepileptic
Chloral hydrate	Noctec	Sedative, Hypnotic
Chlordiazepoxide	Librium	Antianxiety
Chlormezanone	Trancopal	Antianxiety
Chlorpromazine	Thorazine	Antipsychotic
Chlorprothixene	Taractan	Antipsychotic
Clomipramine	Not Approved	Antidepressant
Clonazepam	Clonopin	Antiepileptic
Clonidine	Catapres	Antihypertensive
Clorazepate	Tranxene	Antianxiety
Cyproheptadine	Periactin	Antiasthmatic
Dantrolene sodium	Dantrium	Skeletal muscle relaxant
Deanol	Deaner	Stimulant
Desipramine	Norpramin, Pertofrane	Antidepressant
Desmethylimipramine	Not Approved	Antidepressant
Dextroamphetamine sulfate	Dexedrine	Stimulant
Diazepam	Valium	Antiepileptic, Skeletal muscle relaxant, Antianxiety

Appendix C—Continued

Generic Name	Trade Name*	Classification
Diphenhydramine	Benadryl	Sedative, Hypnotic, Antihistamine
Diphenylhydantoin sodium	Dilantin	Antiepileptic
Doxepin	Adapin, Sinequan	Antidepressant
Ethchlorvynol	Placidyl	Sedative, Hypnotic
Ethinamate	Valmid	Sedative, Hypnotic
Ethopropazine	Parsidol	Anticholinergic, Antiparkinsonism
Ethosuximide	Zarontin	Antiepileptic
Ethotoin	Peganone	Antiepileptic
Fenfluramine	Pondimin	Anorectic
Fluphenazine	Prolixin, Permitil	Antipsychotic
Flurazepam	Dalmane	Sedative, Hypnotic
Glutethimide	Doriden	Sedative, Hypnotic
Halazepam	Paxipam	Antianxiety
Haloperidol	Haldol	Antipsychotic
Hydroxyzine	Atarax, Vistaril, Durrax	Sedative, Hypnotic, Antianxiety
Imipramine	Janimine, SK-Pramine, Tofranil	Antidepressant
Isocarboxazid	Marplan	Antidepressant
Levoamphetamine	Not Approved	Stimulant
Lithium carbonate	Eskalith, Lithane, Lithonate	Antipsychotic
Lorazepam	Ativan	Antianxiety
Loxapine	Loxitane	Antipsychotic
Mephenytoin	Mesantoin	Antiepileptic
Mephobarbital	Mebaral	Antiepileptic
Meprobamate	Miltown, Equanil	Antianxiety
Mesoridazine	Serentil	Antipsychotic
Methamphetamine	Desoxyn	Stimulant
Methaqualone	Quaalude, Sopor	Sedative, Hypnotic
Metharbital	Gemonil	Antiepileptic
Methotrimeprazine	Levoprome	Antipsychotic
Methsuximide	Celontin	Antiepileptic
Methylphenidate	Ritalin	Stimulant
Methyprylon	Noludar	Sedative, Hypnotic
Molindone	Moban	Antipsychotic
Nortriptyline	Aventyl, Pamelor	Antidepressant
Oxazepam	Serax	Antianxiety
Paramethadione	Paradione	Antiepileptic
Pemoline	Cylert	Stimulant
Penfluridol	Not Approved	Antipsychotic

Appendix C—Continued

Generic Name	Trade Name*	Classification
Pentobarbital	Nembutal	Sedative, Hypnotic
Perphenazine	Trilafon	Antipsychotic
Phenacemide	Phenurone	Antiepileptic
Phenelzine	Nardil	Antidepressant
Phenobarbital	Luminal	Antiepileptic, Sedative, Hypnotic
Phensuximide	Milontin	Antiepileptic
Phenytoin	Dilantin	Antiepileptic
Pimozide	Orap	Antipsychotic
Piperacetazine	Quide	Antipsychotic
Piracetam	Not Approved	Nootropic
Parzepam	Centrax, Verstron	Antianxiety
Primidone	Mysoline	Antiepileptic
Prochlorperazine	Compazine	Antipsychotic
Procyclidine	Kemadrin	Anticholinergic, Antiparkinsonism
Promazine	Sparine	Antipsychotic
Promethazine	Phenergan	Sedative, Hypnotic
Propranolol	Inderal	Beta-Adrenergic Blocker
Protriptyline	Vivactil	Antidepressant
Reserpine	Serpasil	Antipsychotic
Secobarbital	Seconal	Sedative, Hypnotic
Temazepam	Restoril	Sedative, Hypnotic
Thioridazine	Mellaril	Antipsychotic
Thiothixene	Navane	Antipsychotic
Tranylcypromine	Parnate	Antidepressant
Trazodone	Desyrel	Antidepressant
Triazolam	Halcion	Sedative, Hypnotic
Thiethylperazine	Torecan	Antipsychotic
Trifluoperazine	Stelazine	Antipsychotic
Triflupromazine	Vesprin	Antipsychotic
Trihexyphenidyl	Artane	Anticholinergic, Antiparkinsonism
Trimethadione	Tridione	Antiepileptic
Trimipramine	Surmontil	Antidepressant
Valproic acid	Depakene	Antiepileptic

*In the case of drugs no longer protected by patent laws, the inclusion of trade names other than the original was arbitrary. Not apoproved = drugs not approved for general use by the Food and Drug Administration (FDA) as of 1984.

APPENDIX D

Alphabetical List of Selected Psychotropic and Antiepileptic Drugs by Trade Name (United States) With Corresponding Generic Name

Trade Name	Generic Name	Trade Name	Generic Name
Adapin	Doxepin	Elavil	Amitriptyline
Akineton	Biperiden	Endep	Amitriptyline
Alurate	Aprobarbital	Equanil	Meprobamate
Artane	Trihexylphenidyl	Eskalith	Lithium carbonate
Asendin	Amoxapine		
Atabrine	Quinacrine	Gemonil	Metharbital
Atarax	Hydroxyzine		
Ativan	Lorazepam	Halcion	Triazolam
Aventyl	Nortriptyline	Haldol	Haloperidol
Benadryl	Diphenhydramine	Inderal	Propranolol
Benzedrine	Amphetamine		
Butisol	Butabarbital	Janimine	Imipramine
Catapres	Clonidine	Kemadrin	Procyclidine
Celontin	Methsuximide		
Centrax	Prazepam	Levoprome	Methotrimeprazine
Clonopin	Clonazepam	Librium	Chlordiazepoxide
Cogentin	Benztropine	Lithane	Lithium carbonate
Compazine	Prochlorperazine	Lithonate	Lithium carbonate
Cylert	Pemoline	Loxitane	Loxapine
		Luminal	Phenobarbital
Dalmane	Flurazepam		
Dantrium	Dantrolene sodium	Marplan	Isocarboxazid
Deaner	Deanol	Mebaral	Mephobarbital
Depakene	Valproic acid	Mellaril	Thioridazine
Desoxyn	Methamphetamine	Meprospan	Meprobamate
Desyrel	Trazodone	Mesantoin	Mephenytoin
Dexedrine	Dextroamphetamine	Milontin	Phensuximide
Diamox	Acetazolamide	Miltown	Meprobamate
Dilantin	Phenytoin	Moban	Molindone
Doriden	Glutethimide	Mysoline	Primidone
Durrax	Hydroxyzine		

Appendix D—Continued

Trade Name	Generic Name	Trade Name	Generic Name
Nardil	Phenelzine	Seconal	Secobarbital
Navane	Thiothixene	Serax	Oxazepam
Nembutal	Pentobarbital	Serentil	Mesoridazine
Noctec	Chloral hydrate	Serpasil	Reserpine
Noludar	Methyprylon	Sinequan	Doxepin
Norpramin	Desipramine	SK-Pramine	Imipramine
		Sopor	Methaqualone
		Sparine	Promazine
Orap	Pimozide	Stelazine	Trifluoperazine
		Surmontil	Trimipramine
		Symmetrel	Amantadine
Pamelor	Nortriptyline		
Paradione	Paramethadione	Taractan	Chlorprothixene
Parnate	Tranylcypromine	Tegretol	Carbamazepine
Parsidol	Ethopropazine	Thorazine	Chlorpromazine
Paxipam	Halazepam	Tindal	Acetophenazine
Peganone	Ethotoin	Tofranil	Imipramine
Periactin	Cyproheptadine	Torecan	Thiethylperazine
Permitil	Fluphenazine	Trancopal	Chlormezanone
Pertofrane	Desipramine	Tranxene	Clorazepate
Phenergan	Promethazine	Tridione	Trimethadione
Phenurone	Phenacemide	Trilafon	Perphenazine
Placidyl	Ethchlorvynol		
Pondimin	Fenfluramine	Valium	Diazepam
Prolixin	Fluphenazine	Valmid	Ethinamate
		Vesprin	Triflupromazine
		Vistaril	Hydroxyzine pamoate
Quaalude	Methaqualone	Vivactil	Protriptyline
Quide	Piperacetazine		
		Xanax	Alprazolam
Restoril	Temazepam		
Ritalin	Methylphenidate	Zarontin	Ethosuximide

APPENDIX E

Dyskinesia Identification System—Coldwater (DIS-Co)

NAME: _____

HOSPITAL NUMBER: _____

HOUSEHOLD: _____

DATE: _____

TIME: _____ AM PM RATER: _____

I. FACIAL:
   1. Tics ....0 1 2 3 4 NA
   2. Grimaces ....0 1 2 3 4 NA
   a. Other ....0 1 2 3 4 NA

II. OCULAR:
   3. Biopharospasm ....0 1 2 3 4 NA
   4. Blinking ....0 1 2 3 4 NA
   b. Other ....0 1 2 3 4 NA

III. ORAL:
   5. Lip Smacking ....0 1 2 3 4 NA
   6. Pursing/Puckering ....0 1 2 3 4 NA
   7. Sucking ....0 1 2 3 4 NA
   8. Upper Lip Tremor ....0 1 2 3 4 NA
   9. Thrusting Lower Lip ....0 1 2 3 4 NA
  10. Cheek Puffing ....0 1 2 3 4 NA
  11. Chewing ....0 1 2 3 4 NA
  12. Lateral Jaw ....0 1 2 3 4 NA
   c. Other ....0 1 2 3 4 NA

IV. LINGUAL:
  13. Clonic Tongue ....0 1 2 3 4 NA
  14. Tonic Tongue ....0 1 2 3 4 NA
  15. Tongue Thrusts ....0 1 2 3 4 NA
  16. Tongue in Cheek ....0 1 2 3 4 NA
  17. Tongue Tremors ....0 1 2 3 4 NA

18. Lateral Tongue	0	1	2	3	4	NA
19. Myokymic Tongue	0	1	2	3	4	NA
20. Athetoid Tongue	0	1	2	3	4	NA
d. Other	0	1	2	3	4	NA

V. HEAD/NECK:

21. Retrocollis	0	1	2	3	4	NA
22. Torticollis	0	1	2	3	4	NA
e. Other	0	1	2	3	4	NA

VI. TRUNK:

23. Axial Hyperkinesia	0	1	2	3	4	NA
24. Shoulder/Hip Torsion	0	1	2	3	4	NA
f. Other	0	1	2	3	4	NA

VII. UPPER LIMB:

25. Myokymic Finger/Wrist/Arm	0	1	2	3	4	NA
26. Athetoid Finger/Wrist/Arm	0	1	2	3	4	NA
27. Pill Rolling	0	1	2	3	4	NA
28. Finger Counting	0	1	2	3	4	NA
g. Other	0	1	2	3	4	NA

VIII. LOWER LIMB:

29. Walking in Place	0	1	2	3	4	NA
30. Foot Tapping	0	1	2	3	4	NA
31. Ankle Flexion	0	1	2	3	4	NA
32. Toe Movement	0	1	2	3	4	NA
h. Other	0	1	2	3	4	NA

IX. GROSS BODY:

33. Holokinetic	0	1	2	3	4	NA
i. Other	0	1	2	3	4	NA

X. AMBULATORY:

34. Gait	0	1	2	3	4	NA
j. Other	0	1	2	3	4	NA

0—NOT PRESENT	Abnormal movements are *not observed*. Some movements may be observed but are not considered abnormal.
1—MINIMAL	Abnormal movements occur *infrequently and/or* are *difficult to detect*.
2—MILD	Abnormal movements occur *infrequently and are easy to detect*.
3—MODERATE	Abnormal movements occur *frequently and are easy to detect*.
4—SEVERE	Abnormal movements occur *almost continuously and/or are of extreme intensity*.
NA—NOT ASSESSED	The rater is not able to make an assessment.

Note. "From The Dyskinesia Identification System—Coldwater (DIS-Co): A Tardive Dyskinesia Rating Scale for the Developmentally Disabled." By R. L. Sprague et al., 1984, *Psychopharmacology Bulletin, 20*, p. 329. Reprinted by permission.

APPENDIX F

DIS-Co Item Identification

I. Facial Movements

1. Tics — Brief, muscular contractions of small sections of the face.
2. Grimaces — Brief, muscular contractions of large sections of the face.
a. Other

II. Ocular Movements

3. Blepharospasm — Fine tremors of the eyelid(s)
4. Blinking — Rapid opening and closing of the eyelids.

III. Oral Movements

5. Lip Smacking — Quick parting of the lips, which may produce a smacking sound.
6. Pursing — Puckering of the lips.
7. Sucking — Drawing in of lips, cheeks, air, etc., caused by lip-tongue action.
8. Upper Lip Tremor — Quivering of the upper lip (Rabbit syndrome).
9. Thrusting of the Lower Lip — Extending the lower lip similar to a child's pout.
10. Cheek Puffing — Forcing air into the cheeks producing a noticeable bulge.
11. Chewing — Circular or up and down jaw movements (similar to movements that occur during eating).
12. Lateral Jaw Movement — Side-to-side movement of the jaw.

IV. Lingual Movements

13. Clonic Tongue — Rhythmic movement of the tongue in and out of the mouth
14. Tonic Tongue Protrusion — Extending the tongue and holding beyond the lips.
15. Tongue Thrusts — Abruptly moving the tongue in and out of the mouth.
16. Tongue in Cheek — Tongue pressed against the inside of the cheeks or lips, producing a noticeable bulge.

17. Tongue Tremors	Quivering of the tongue, observed with the mouth open and tongue resting inside or outside the mouth.
18. Lateral Tongue	Side-to-side movements of the tongue inside the mouth.
19. Myokymic Tongue Movements	Twitching movements of sections of the tongue, observed with the mouth open and tongue resting inside the mouth.
20. Athetoid Tongue Movements	Worm-like rolling and twisting movements.

V. Head/Neck Movements

21. Retrocollis	Contractions of the muscles in the back of the neck which results in the head being tilted back.
22. Torticollis	Contractions of the neck muscles twisting the head to one side (similar to a stiff neck).

VI. Trunk Movements

23. Axial Hyperkinesia	Front to back or circular movements of the pelvis.
24. Shoulder/Hip Torsion	Twisting, rolling movements of the shoulders and/or hips, involving large sections of the body.

VII. Upper Limb Movements

25. Myokymic Finger/Wrist/Arm	Twitching movements observed of the fingers, wrists, and/or arms.
26. Athetoid Finger/Wrist/Arm	Worm-like rolling and twisting movements observed in the fingers, wrists, and/or arms.
27. Pill Rolling	Circular movements of the thumb against the fingers of the same hand.
28. Finger Counting	Tapping of the thumb against the fingers of the same hand.

VIII. Lower Limb Movements

29. Walking in Place	Alternating from one foot to the other while standing.
30. Foot Tapping	An alternating heel-toe tapping or striking of the floor with the entire foot, heel, and/or toe.
31. Ankle Flexion	Circular, up and down and/or back and forth bending movements of the ankle.
32. Toe Movement	Movements or bending of the toe(s).

IX. Gross Body Movements

33. Holokinetic	Sudden, unexpected, clumsy movements of large sections of the body.

X. Ambulatory Movements

34. Gait	Shuffling of the feet while walking may be accompanied by arm extension and/or bent knees.

Note. "From The Dyskinesia Identification System-Coldwater (DIS-Co): A Tardive Dyskinesia Rating Scale for the Developmentally Disabled," by R. L. Sprague et al., 1984, *Psychopharmacology Bulletin, 20,* p. 329. Reprinted by permission.

APPENDIX G

Dyskinesia Identification System: Condensed User Scale (DISCUS)

NAME: _____

ID #: _____

UNIT: _____

DATE: _____

TIME: START _____ STOP _____ AM/PM

RATER: _____

COOPERATION LEVEL (circle one):

1 : NO CO-OP (passive or active resistance; few, if any, examination steps done)

2 : PARTIAL CO-OP (at least one activation task done; some but not all examination steps)

3 : FULL CO-OP (most or all examination steps)

FACIAL:
1. Tics ....0 1 2 3 4 NA
2. Grimaces............0 1 2 3 4 NA

OCULAR:
3. Blinking ....0 1 2 3 4 NA

ORAL:
4. Chewing/Lip
   Smacking ....0 1 2 3 4 NA
5. Puckering/Sucking/
   Thrusting Lower
   Lip................0 1 2 3 4 NA

LINGUAL:
6. Tongue Thrusts/
   Tongue in Cheek .....0 1 2 3 4 NA

OTHERS:

_____ 0 1 2 3 4 NA

_____ 0 1 2 3 4 NA

_____ 0 1 2 3 4 NA

_____ 0 1 2 3 4 NA

_____ 0 1 2 3 4 NA

_____ 0 1 2 3 4 NA

COMMENTS:

_____

_____

_____

_____

_____

214

7. Tonic Tongue . . . . .0 1 2 3 4 NA
8. Tongue Tremor . . . . . . .0 1 2 3 4 NA
9. Athetoid/Myokymic/
   Lateral Tongue . . . . . . .0 1 2 3 4 NA

HEAD/NECK/TRUNK:
10. Retrocollis/
    Torticollis . . . . .0 1 2 3 4 NA
11. Shoulder/Hip
    Torsion . . . . .0 1 2 3 4 NA

UPPER LIMB:
12. Athetoid/Myokymic
    Finger-Wrist-Arm
    (not tremor) . . . . .0 1 2 3 4 NA
13. Pill Rolling . . . . .0 1 2 3 4 NA

LOWER LIMB:
14. Ankle Flexion/
    Foot Tapping. . . . . . . .0 1 2 3 4 NA
15. Toe Movement . . . . . . .0 1 2 3 4 NA

SCORING

0—NOT PRESENT (movements not observed or some movements observed but not considered abnormal)

1—MINIMAL (abnormal movements are difficult to detect or movements are easy to detect but occur only once or twice in a short nonrepetitive manner)

2—MILD (abnormal movements occur infrequently and are easy to detect)

3—MODERATE (abnormal movements occur frequently and are easy to detect)

4—SEVERE (abnormal movements occur almost continuously and are easy to detect)

NA—NOT ASSESSED (an assessment for an item is not able to be made)

Note: From "Dyskinesia Identification System: Condensed User Scale (DISCUS)" by R. L. Sprague, J.E. Kalachnik, and D. M. White, 1985, Champaign, IL: Institute for Child Behavior and Development, University of Illinois at Champaign-Urbana. Reprinted by permission.

APPENDIX H

Alphabetical List of Selected United Kingdom Trade Names*

Trade Name	Generic Name	Trade Name	Generic Name
Allegron	nortriptyline	Moditen	fluphenazine
Almazine	lorazepam		
Anafranil	clomipramine	Nozinan	methotrimeprazine
Apsolol	propranolol		
		Phasal	lithium carbonate
Berkoldol	propranolol	Ponderax	fenfluramine
		Priadel	lithium carbonate
Camcolit	lithium carbonate		
		Rivotril	clonazepam
Domical	amitriptyline	Ronyl	pemoline
Emeside	ethosuximide	Serenace	haloperidol
Epanutin	phenytoin	Serenid-D	oxazepam
Epilim	sodium valporate	Serenid Forte	oxazepam
		Soneryl	butabarbitone
Fentazin	perphenazine	Stemetil	prochlorperazine
Fortunan	haloperidol		
		Tryptizol	amitriptyline
Largactil	chlorpromazine		
Lentizol	amitriptyline	Veractil	methotrimeprazine
Liskonum	lithium carbonate	Vertigon	prochlorperazine
		Volital	pemoline
Modecate	fluphenazine		

*Only trade names that are *not* used in the United States are listed.

Glossary

Abbreviated Teacher Rating Scale: a shortened, 10 item version of Conners' 39 Item Teacher Rating Scale (see Appendix B).

abdominal epilepsy: same as autonomic epilepsy.

aberrant: behavior that deviates markedly from what is considered normal.

absence seizure: same as petit mal seizure.

absorption: the process whereby a substance is taken into or across tissues, e.g., intestine; the movement of a drug into the bloodstream.

ACTH: adrenocorticotropic hormone.

acute: having a sudden onset and short duration.

acute dystonic reaction: characterized by uncontrolled muscle activity with stiffness or twisting of body parts; possible reactions include facial grimacing; torticollis, which may be associated with oculogyric crisis; and opisthotonos. A side effect of antipsychotic drugs occasionally seen with the initiation of treatment.

adaptive: having a capacity for modification to fit the demands of the environment.

adrenocorticotropic hormone: a hormone secreted by the anterior lobe of the pituitary gland which controls the secretion of adrenocortical hormones by the adrenal cortices; corticotropin; ACTH.

adverse reaction: same as side effect.

affective: pertaining to feelings or emotions.

affective disorders: characterized by changes in mood as the primary symptoms, e.g., mania, depression.

agitated: motor restlessness and increased activity level in association with anxiety and tension.

agitation: motor restlessness associated with mental distress.

akathisia: characterized by motor restlessness arising from a compulsion to move about; an extrapyramidal syndrome produced by antipsychotic drugs.

akinetic: cessation of movement.

akinetic seizure: a term used inconsistently in the literature to refer to the seizures associated with the Lennox-Gastaut syndrome; head nodding spells. The seizures are brief and typically consist of a sudden, violent jerk, either forward or backward. If the person is standing the associated fall may cause severe, repeated head injury. Defined by The International League Against Epilepsy as "loss of movement without atonia" (Gastaut, 1970).

ambulatory: able to walk.

anemia: below normal number of red blood cells, amount of hemoglobin, or total drug volume.

anorexia: a lack or loss of appetite for food.

anoxia: absence or loss of oxygen.

antianxiety drug: same as minor tranquilizer.

anticholinergic: an agent that alters the effect of acetylcholine in cholinergic synapses; anticholinergic drugs are used in the management of some extra-pyramidal syndromes produced by antipsychotic drugs.

anticonvulsant: an agent that reduces the frequency, magnitude, or duration of convulsions or seizures; antiepileptic.

antidepressant: an agent that prevents or suppresses the symptoms of depression; mood elevating.

antiepileptic: an agent that reduces the frequency, magnitude, or duration of convulsions or seizures; anticonvulsant.

antipsychotic: an agent that prevents or suppresses the symptoms of psychosis; major tranquilizer, neuroleptic.

anxiety: a feeling of uneasiness, apprehension, and fear over an anticipated experience.

ataxia: failure of voluntary muscle coordination; **gait ataxia:** a staggered walk with a wide base.

athetosis: characterized by slow, writhing movements of peripheral parts of the body.

atonic: loss of normal tone; **atonic seizure:** patient suddenly crumples and falls to the floor, muscles remain flaccid during the seizure.

ATRS: Abbreviated Teacher Rating Scale.

atypical febrile convulsion: epileptic convulsion in association with a fever illness.

aura: a warning that precedes an epileptic seizure often manifest as a sensation or motor movement.

autism: a subjective, self centered form of thinking that is not correctable with information from external reality.

automatisms: seemingly purposeful involuntary behavior that is out of context; a manifestation of psychomotor epilepsy; **simple automatisms:** repetitive smacking of lips, chewing, mumbling; **complex automatisms:** undressing, walking about.

autonomic nervous system: the part of the nervous system that regulates the muscles of the heart, smooth muscles, and glands.

autonomic epilepsy: an uncommon form of epilepsy in which seizures may be manifest as gastrointestinal disturbances (abdominal pain, vomiting, nausea, etc.), headache, or other symptoms of autonomic dysfunction; thalamic epilepsy, abdominal epilepsy, epileptic equivalent.

behavior modification: a treatment approach based on a model that views abnormal behavior as being acquired in response to environmental stress and learned and maintained in the same manner as normal behavior. The principles of experimental psychology are emphasized, particularly classical and operant conditioning. The importance of the cognitive mediation of behavior and vicarious and symbolic learning processes, e.g., modeling, is also recognized. Treatment conditions are explicitly stated and therapeutic outcomes are measured objectively.

behavior therapy: same as behavior modification.

benign: having a favorable outcome; not recurring.

benzodiazepines: a category of antianxiety agents (minor tranquilizers) which includes diazepam (Valium), chlordiazepoxide (Librium), and clonazepam (Clonopin).

bilateral: pertaining to both sides.

biotransformation: the chemical alteration of a compound within the body, e.g., the metabolism of a drug by liver microsomal enzymes.

blood-brain barrier: refers not to an anatomical structure but to the fact that the capillaries of the brain prevent certain classes of compounds from entering and affecting brain neurons. A closeknit layer of glial cells surrounds the brain capillaries creating an additional barrier for compounds which are not lipid soluble.

brand name: same as trade name.

butyrophenones: a category of antipsychotic agents (major tranquilizers) which includes haloperidol (Haldol).

cardiovascular: pertaining to the heart and blood vessels.

central nervous system: consisting of the brain and spinal cord.

cerebral palsy: a variety of syndromes, characterized by a disorganization of motor control, that are the result of damage to the motor areas of the brain.

chorea: characterized by continuous, random, uncontrolled contractions of different muscle groups.

chronic: persisting over a long period of time.

clonic: pertaining to a series of alternate muscle contractions and relaxations.

coarse facies: marked by swelling of the lips, thickening of the subcutaneous tissue of the face and scalp, and broadening of the nose; adverse reaction associated with phenytoin (Dilantin) treatment.

cognitive performance: performance on a specified task generally regarded to measure perception, thinking, and remembering.

colic: acute abdominal pain.

combined drug regimen: the simultaneous treatment of two or more disorders with different drugs.

concomitant: accompanying; joined with another.

convulsion: a violent and involuntary contraction or series of contractions of the voluntary muscles.

convulsive disorder: recurrent seizures; epilepsy.

convulsive threshold: the point at which a stimulus, e.g., electrical discharge, produces a convulsion or seizure.

corticotropin: same as adrenocorticotropic hormone.

deinstitutionalization: the transfer of individuals (e.g., mentally retarded, mentally ill) from institutional or residential care to community placement (e.g., half way houses, group homes).

delusions: a false belief that cannot be changed by reason or evidence from the patient's own senses.

depression: a psychiatric disorder characterized by feelings of personal incompetence, listlessness, insomnia, loss of appetite, and psychomotor slowing.

dermatitis: inflammation of the skin.

diphenylmethanes: a category of antianxiety agents (minor tranquilizers) which includes hydroxyzine hydrochloride (Atarax) and hydroxyzine pamoate (Vistaril).

diplopia: double vision.

distribution: the movement of drug molecules in the bloodstream to the site of drug action; concentration of drug molecules in body compartments.

diuretic: an agent that promotes the secretion of urine.

dose: amount of medication administered.

double blind: characterizing a study of a particular treatment, e.g., drug, in which neither the person administering (evaluating) or receiving the agent is aware of whether the active or inactive (placebo) drug is being given.

drug: any substance other than food that has an effect on living tissue.

drug addiction: "A behavioral pattern of compulsive drug use, characterized by overwhelming involvement with the use of a drug, the securing of its supply, and a high tendency to relapse after withdrawal" (Jaffe, 1975, p. 285).

drug free period: a break in a chronic drug regimen for a period of time during which no medication is administered; drug holiday.

drug holiday: same as drug free period.

drug interaction: the modification of the effects of a drug by the prior or concurrent administration of another drug.

drug of (first) choice: the agent to be administered first in the treatment of a specific disorder, usually determined on the basis of safety and efficacy.

dysarthria: imperfect articulation of speech; slurred speech.

dyskinesia: fragmentary or incomplete movements that result from a diminished power to control voluntary movements.

dysphoria: disquiet; restlessness; malaise.

dystonia: disordered muscle tone.

early infantile autism: a rare disorder with onset during early infancy and characterized by autistic aloneness, absence of language or developmental language disorders, insistence on sameness, repetitive behaviors, and lack of demonstrable physical defect.

echolalia: the repetition of words spoken by other people as if echoing what is said.

edema: swelling resulting from an accumulation of fluid in subcutaneous tissues.

educable mentally retarded: an educational classification for children whose IQs range from 50 or 55 to 75 or 80.

EEG: electroencephalogram.

efficacy: effectiveness.

endocrine system: the glands and structures that produce hormones which are released into the blood.

endoplasmic reticulum: ultramicroscopic network of tubules and cavities within almost all cells; microenzymes in the endoplasmic reticulum of liver cells break drugs down into metabolites that are more easily removed from the body.

enteric-coated: a special coating applied to tablets and capsules that delays absorption until the drug reaches the intestine.

enuresis: involuntary discharge of urine.

enzyme: a protein that brings about or accelerates chemical reactions.

epidemiology: the study of the factors that influence the incidence, distribution, and control of disease.

epilepsy: recurrent seizures that are due to sudden electrical discharges in the brain.

epileptic equivalent: same as autonomic epilepsy.

epileptic seizure precipitated by fever: form of epilepsy characterized by seizures that are triggered by a fever illness.

equilibrium: a state of balance between two opposing forces.

etiology: the causes of a disease; the study of the factors that cause disease.

exacerbate: to make more severe or violent.

excretion: the elimination or discharge of substances, e.g., wastes, metabolites, from the cell, tissue, and blood; drugs are often excreted as water soluble metabolites by the kidney.

extensor: a muscle that extends a joint.

extracellular fluid: fluid outside the cell.

extrapyramidal syndromes: a group of disorders characterized by abnormal involuntary movements. Extrapyramidal syndromes produced by antipsychotic drugs include Parkinsonian syndrome, akathisia, acute dystonic reaction, and tardive dyskinesia.

extrapyramidal tract: not an anatomical structure, but a group of nuclei (a nucleus is a mass of nerve cells) and fibers that control and coordinate motor activities, especially gross intentional movements, patterns of movement, walking movements, and "background" muscle tone.

FDA: Food and Drug Administration.

febrile: relating to or characterized by fever.

Feingold diet: same as Kaiser-Permanente diet.

flexor: any muscle that bends a joint.

focal epilepsy: characterized by seizures associated with an abnormal electrical discharge originating in, or restricted to, a limited area of the brain.

folic acid: substance used by the bone marrow to form red blood cells.

gastrointestinal: pertaining to the stomach and intestines.

generalized seizures: seizures associated with abnormal electrical discharges that affect the entire brain; they may be focal at the onset and spread to become generalized or be generalized from the beginning. Grand mal, petit mal, and myoclonic seizures are all generalized seizures.

generic name: a drug name, not protected by a patent, that identifies a specific chemical structure; official name, nonproprietary name.

Gilles de la Tourette's syndrome: a rare disorder with an onset in childhood characterized by tics, particularly of the facial muscles, and involuntary vocalizations.

gingival hyperplasia: an excessive growth of gum tissue with a mulberry shaped appearance. Irritants lodged in the tissue cause secondary inflammation resulting in a red or bluish-red discoloration. This is an adverse reaction commonly associated with phenytoin (Dilantin).

gonadotropic hormones: Three hormones secreted by the anterior pituitary that have an influence on the ovaries and testes.

grand mal epilepsy: characterized by periodic attacks of unconsciousness and generalized tonic and clonic movements frequently lasting from 3 to 5 minutes. Interseizure EEG findings may be normal and seizures can begin at any age. Generalized seizures fall into four categories: Tonic-clonic, clonic, tonic, and atonic.

growth rebound: an increase in growth rate following the cessation of stimulant drug treatment in hyperactive children.

hallucination: perception of an object in the absence of corresponding stimuli.

hallucinogens: a category of psychotropic drugs capable of inducing hallucinations.

hirsutism: abnormal hairiness; an adverse drug reaction associated with phenytoin (Dilantin) therapy.

hydantoinates: a category of antiepileptic drugs with potent anticonvulsant properties that includes phenytoin (Dilantin), mephentoin (Mesantoin), and ethotoin (Peganone).

hyperactivity: a long term, persistent behavior disorder characterized by excessive restlessness and inattentiveness originating during early to middle childhood (2 to 6 years of age).

hypertonicity: characterized by excessive skeletal muscle tone; the muscle is more resistant to passive stretching.

hypnotic: a category of psychotropic drugs that induce sleep.

hypoplasia: failure of an organ to develop and reach its adult size.

hypotension: abnormally low blood pressure.

hypothalamic epilepsy: same as autonomic epilepsy.

hypsarrythmia: an exceedingly abnormal electroencephalographic pattern between seizures characterized by random, high voltage slow waves and spikes that originate from multiple foci and spread to all cortical areas. This EEG pattern is associated with myoclonic epilepsy of young children (infantile spasms, salaam seizures, massive myoclonia). Severe mental retardation is common.

idiopathic: a disease of spontaneous origin or unknown cause.

incidence: the number of new cases, e.g., of a disease, during a certain period of time.

infantile spasms: same as myoclonic epilepsy of young children.

induce: to bring about by stimulation; cause something to occur.

insomnia: inability to sleep.

intracellular fluid: fluid within the cell.

intractable: resistant to control.

intramuscular: within the substance of the muscle.

intravenous: within a vein.

in utero: within the uterus.

Isle of Wight: island of the southern coast of England.

Jacksonian seizure: a focal seizure characterized by unilateral clonic movements that start in one group of muscles moving systematically to adjacent groups of muscles. The seizures are due to an abnormal electrical discharge that originates in, and spreads across, the motor cortex.

jaundice: a syndrome characterized by an excess of bile pigment in the blood and yellow appearance of the skin resulting from the deposition of bile pigments in the skin; icterus.

Kaiser-Permanente diet: a treatment regimen for childhood behavior disorders, especially hyperactivity, which involves the elimination of low molecular weight chemicals, e.g., salicylates and artificial colors and additives, from daily food intake; K-P diet, Feingold diet.

ketogenic diet: a dietary regimen in which the total daily consumption of fat. (in grams) is at least four times greater than proteins and carbohydrates combined (in grams). This maintains the state of ketosis achieved by a marked reduction in food intake at the onset of treatment. The diet is effective in treating myoclonic epilepsy in young children.

kg: kilogram.

kilogram: a unit of weight in the metric system being 1000 grams; equivalent to approximately 2.2 pounds.

K-P diet: same as Kaiser-Permanente diet.

learning performance: performance on a specified task generally regarded to measure learning rather than a more pure measure of the neural events associated with learning.

least restrictive alternative: handicapped children, including children in public and private institutions, are educated as much as possible with children who are not handicapped. Separate schools, special classes, or other removal of any handicapped child from the regular program is appropriate only if the regular educational environment accompanied by supplementary aids and services is not adequate to give the child what he or she needs.

Lennox-Gastaut syndrome: one type of myoclonic epilepsy characterized by several types of seizures including staring spells, myoclonic seizures (sudden violent jerks with an associated fall, sudden falls without jerks, head nodding seizures, and sagging attacks (atonic seizures), and generalized tonic-clonic seizures. Age of onset is usually between 3 to 5 years of age. Mental and motor retardation are common. Interseizure EEG findings often show modified hypsarrhythmia (2 per second spike and wave). Also called petit mal variant, myoclonic epilepsy of older children.

lipids: a group of substances, such as fatty acids, that cannot be dissolved in water. Lipids are stored in the body, are used as fuel, and are an important part of all living cells.

lipid soluble: capable of being dissolved in lipids.

mainstreaming: an approach to the delivery of special education services that emphasizes the integration of the handicapped child with nonhandicapped peers in regular classrooms as opposed to segregation in self contained special classes. The educational needs of the child are met through modifications in the regular school program.

major motor epilepsy: same as grand mal epilepsy.

major tranquilizer: a category of psychotropic drugs that includes the phenothiazines, thiozanthenes, and butyrophenones; antipsychotic agents, neuroleptics. These drugs are used primarily in the treatment of psychotic disorders.

maladaptive: not promoting or assisting adaptation.

malaise: an indefinite feeling of bodily discomfort or lack of health.

MAO inhibitor: same as monamine oxidase inhibitor.

massive myoclonic seizures: same as myoclonic epilepsy of young children.

mcg: microgram.

μcg: microgram.

mcg/ml: microgram per milliliter.

μcg/ml: microgram per milliliter.

MCT: medium chain triglycerides.

megavitamins: massive doses of vitamins. A treatment of questionable efficacy for learning disabilities, hyperactivity, adult psychosis, and convulsions consisting of large doses of niacin, niacinamide, ascorbic acid, pyridoxine, and calcium pantothenate or other vitamins either individually or in combination. Possibly effective in the treatment of childhood psychosis.

mental retardation: "Significantly subaverage general intellectual functioning existing concurrently with deficits in adaptive behavior, and manifested during the developmental period" (Grossman, 1973, p. 11). Classification according to the severity of symptoms (IQ score) is as follows: mild (55–69), moderate (40–54), severe (25–39), and profound (below 25). The terms *borderline, dull-normal* and *slow learning* are occasionally used to refer to children with IQ's from 70 to 89.

metabolism: the sum of the processes in the building up and maintenance of living substance and the production of energy for vital activities; the sum of the processes by which the body transforms a substance, e.g., drug.

metabolite: any substance produced by a metabolic process.

mg: milligram.

mg/kg: milligram per kilogram.

microgram: a unit of weight in the metric system being one one-millionth of a gram or one one-thousandth of a milligram.

microsomal enzymes: enzymes within the cells of the liver that participate in the metabolism of many drugs.

migraine: a condition marked by periodic attacks of severe headaches often associated with nausea and vomiting. The attacks are preceded by constriction of cranial arteries and begin with the dilation of the arteries.

milligram: a unit of weight in the metric system being one one-thousandth of a gram; equivalent to approximately one twenty-eight thousandth of an ounce.

milliliter: a metric unit of capacity being one one-thousandth of a liter.

minimal brain dysfunction: a syndrome found "in children of near average, average, or above average general intelligence" and characterized by "learning or behavioral disabilities ranging from mild to severe, which are associated with deviations of function of the central nervous system. These deviations may manifest themselves by various combinations of impairment in perception, conceptualization, language, memory, and control of attention, impulse, or motor function . . ." (Clements, 1966, p. 9–10).

minor tranquilizer: a category of psychotropic drugs with sedative and antianxiety properties which includes the benzodiazepines, propanediol carbamates, and hydroxyzine.

mixed epilepsy: two or more different types of epilepsy manifest at the same time.

ml: milliliter.

monoamine oxidase inhibitor: a category of antidepressant drugs that includes tranylcypromine (Parnate) and phenelzine (Nardil),

motor cortex: the area of the brain that controls discrete movements of the skeletal muscles.

muscle tone: a slight degree of muscle tension produced by continuous neural stimulation.

mutism: inability or refusal to speak.

myoclonic epilepsy: consists of several different types of epilepsy including myoclonic epilepsy of young children (infantile spasms, West syndrome) and myoclonic epilepsy of older children (Lennox-Gastaut syndrome, petit mal variant), both of which appear to be the same disorder but with different age at onset of seizures. Classification of the other types of myoclonic epilepsy is incomplete but includes children and adolescents with myoclonic seizures who do not manifest the symptoms associated with infantile spasms or the Lennox-Gastaut syndrome.

myoclonic epilepsy of older children: same as Lennox-Gastaut syndrome.

myoclonic epilepsy of young children: characterized by brief (several seconds) myoclonic seizures that usually occur in clusters lasting several minutes and abnormal interseizure EEG findings called hypsarhythmia. Onset of seizures is commonly between 3 and 9 months of age. Severe mental retardation is common. Also called infantile spasms, West syndrome.

myoclonic seizure: flexor spasm of the musculature; extensor spasms much less common.

narcolepsy: a condition characterized by an uncontrollable desire to sleep or periodic attacks of deep sleep.

neuroleptic: same as antipsychotic agent.

neuropharmacology: the branch of pharmacology that investigates the effects of drugs on the nervous system.

nocturnal: pertaining to night.

nonproprietary name: same as generic name.

nystagmus: a rapid involuntary movement of the eyeball either horizontally, vertically, or in a rotatory manner.

oculogyric crisis: fixed upward gaze; a symptom associated with acute dystonic reaction, an extrapyramidal syndrome produced by some antipsychotic drugs.

official name: same as generic name.

opiates: a group of drugs consisting of opium and its derivatives.

opisthotonos: a type of muscle spasm in which the back is arched, head and heels are bent backward, and the body bowed forward.

organic: pertaining to, or arising from, the organs; affecting the structure of an organism.

organic epilepsy: epilepsy that develops subsequent to permanent, nonprogressive damage to the brain, e.g., head trauma, brain infections.

orthopedic: pertainint to the correction of musculoskeletal deformities; marked by crippling.

orthostatic hypotension: weakness or fainting on rising to an erect position.

osteomalacia: a condition that results from vitamin D and calcium deficiency characterized by softening of the bones, pain, anorexia, and muscular weakness.

oxazolidinediones: a category of antiepileptic drugs that include trimethadione (Tridione) and paramethadione (Paradione).

panic anxiety: a psychiatric disorder characterized by recurrent and unexplained panic attacks with feelings of impending doom. The attacks may be associated with physical symptoms such as breathing difficulties or heart palpitations.

Parkinsonian syndrome: an extra-pyramidal syndrome characterized by psychomotor slowing, masklike facial expression, shuffling gait without free swing of the arms, rigidity, and tremor. "Pill rolling" movements may also be present. An adverse reaction associated with antipsychotic drug therapy.

parenteral: administration by a route other than the digestive tract; any of several routes of injection including subcutaneous, intramuscular, and intravenous.

pathognomonic: characteristic of a disease; a sign or symptom that is used to make a diagnosis.

pathology: the study of the structural and functional changes in tissues and organs of the body that are caused by disease; deviations from the normal that characterize disease.

pediatric psychopharmacology: the branch of pharmacology that investigates the behavioral effects of drugs in children.

petit mal epilepsy: characterized by periodic attacks of altered consciousness usually lasting from 5 to 30 seconds. The seizure is manifest as a sudden cessation of movement and vacant staring into space. In some children the eyes roll back into the head. Seizures may be associated with brief clonic movements that usually recur at a frequency of 3 per second or automatisms. An EEG finding of 3 per second spike-wave forms is pathognomonic of petit mal epilepsy; absence epilepsy.

petit mal variant: same as Lennox-Gastaut syndrome.

pharmacology: the science that deals with the chemical properties, biochemical and physiological effects, absorption, distribution, biotransformation, excretion and therapeutic uses of drugs.

pharmacotherapy: the treatment of disease with medicines.

phenothiazines: a group of antipsychotic drugs which includes chlorpromazine (Thorazine) and thioridazine (Mellaril).

phobia: a persistent abnormal fear.

photophobia: abnormal intolerance to light.

photosensitivity: abnormal reaction of the skin to sunlight.

pigmentation: an abnormal increase of coloration by melanin.

pill rolling: as if rolling a pill between the fingers; a symptom of Parkinsonian syndrome.

placebo: an inactive medication administered to satisfy a patient's need for drug therapy; an inert substance used to control for expectancy effects in pharmacological research; a procedure with no intrinsic therapeutic value.

polypharmacy: the simultaneous administration of two or more drugs.

post seizure phenomena: disturbances following the active stages of a seizure including weakness, nausea, fatigue, muscle soreness, headache, irritability, confusion, and abnormal behavior.

post seizure sleep: period of deep sleep following a seizure.

prevalence: total number of cases in a specific area during a certain period of time.

prolonged seizure: an individual seizure lasting for an uncharacteristically long time.

propanediols: a group of antianxiety agents that includes meprobamate (Equanil, Miltown); propanediol carbamates.

prophylaxis: preventive treatment.

proteins: any one of a group of complex compounds consisting of a combination of amino acids; the principal constituents of all living cells.

psychic seizures: a type of psychomotor seizure manifest as changes in perception, thought, self awareness, mood, or affect.

psychomotor: relating to muscular actions resulting from conscious mental activity.

psychomotor epilepsy: characterized by periodic attacks of altered consciousness lasting from one to several minutes. Seizures may be manifest as a cessation of movement starting with or without automatisms or as changes in perception, thought, self awareness, mood, or affect. EEG findings usually show interseizure temporal lobe abnormalities. Also called temporal lobe epilepsy or complex partial seizure disorders.

psychomotor slowing: manifest as an inability to respond spontaneously at a normal speed, weak voice and labored speech, deliberate body movements, fixed facial expression, and a slowed, dragging walk.

psychopathology: mental disorders; the study of such dysfunctions.

psychopharmacology: the branch of pharmacology that investigates the effects of drugs on behavior.

psychosis: a general term for any severe mental disorder involving a loss of contact with reality and usually associated with delusions, hallucinations, or illusions.

psychotropic drug: any agent that has its principal effect on mood, thought processes, or behavior; behavior modifying drug.

rebound effect: reaction to the withdrawal of medication that may be manifested as an aggravation of the symptoms of the disorder being treated.

refractory: unresponsive to treatment.

relapse: a return of a disease after it apparently ceased.

remission: the lessening or cessation of the symptoms of a disease.

rickets: a condition that results from vitamin D deficiency characterized by bending or distortion of the bones.

salicylates: a group of drugs with analgesic, fever reducing, and anti-inflammatory properties, e.g., aspirin.

schizophrenia: a psychotic disorder characterized by emotional distortion, ambivalence, disturbances of thought, retreat from reality, delusions, hallucinations, and withdrawn or bizarre behavior.

secondary epilepsy: same as organic epilepsy.

sedative: a category of psychotropic drugs that reduce excitement and having a calming effect.

seizure: a sudden attack; fit. **Epileptic seizure:** a loss or alteration of consciousness associated with involuntary muscle movement (or cessation of movement) and abnormal electrical discharges in the brain; convulsion, spell, fit.

self limiting: limited by its own nature and not by outside influences. Self limiting side effects run a limited course and terminate on their own.

separation anxiety: apprehension resulting from loss of contact with significant persons or familiar surroundings; common in infants 6 to 10 months old.

serial grand mal (major motor) seizures: characterized by recurrent grand mal seizures during which the person regains consciousness between attacks; frequently associated with the abrupt withdrawal of antiepileptic medication.

side effect: a consequence other than that for which an agent or treatment is being used; adverse reaction, toxic effects, untoward reaction.

simple febrile seizure: a benign, nonepileptic disorder characterized by brief generalized seizures that occur usually 2 to 6 hours after the onset of a fever. The disorder rarely lasts beyond 6 years of age.

spasm: a sudden and involuntary muscle contraction.

spasticity: increase over normal muscle tone; hypertonicity.

sphincter: a muscle that forms a ring around a body opening, e.g., urethra, and prevents passage via constriction.

spontaneous: occuring without external influence; voluntary.

status epilepticus: a series of seizures in succession during which the person does not regain consciousness between attacks; usually refers to grand mal status.

status seizure: a series of recurring seizures during which the patient does not regain consciousness between seizures.

stereotypic behavior: repetitive and often bizarre motor movements such as rhythmic rocking, head weaving, hand or arm flapping, and rubbing parts of the body; stereotypies.

stereotypies: same as stereotypic behavior.

stimulant: a category of psychotropic drugs that includes methylphenidate (Ritalin), dextroamphetamine (Dexedrine) and pemoline (Cylert).

subcutaneous: beneath the skin.

succinimides: a category of antiepileptic drugs particularly effective in the treatment of petit mal epilepsy that includes ethosuximide (Zarontin), methsuximide (Celontin), and phensuximide (Milontin).

symptomatic epilepsy: seizures are one of the symptoms of a specific disorder that involves the brain, e.g., cerebral degenerative disease.

syndrome: a set of symptoms that occur together and characterize a specific disorder.

tardive dyskinesia: a late appearing extrapyramidal syndrome characterized by involuntary, repetitive movements usually in the region of the mouth but may involve the limbs and trunk as well. Movements include tongue protrusion, licking or smacking of the lips, side to side movements of the chin, blowing of the cheeks, facial grimacing, and eye blinking. A side effect of long term antipsychotic drug treatment.

temporal lobe epilepsy: same as psychomotor epilepsy.

thiozanthenes: a category of antipsychotic agents that includes prothixene (Taractan) and thiothixene (Navane).

teratogen: a substance that causes physical defects in the developing embryo.

tic: spasmodic movement of a muscle; a twitching movement especially of a facial muscle.

titration: a method for determining the strength of a solution or the concentration of a substance in solution, used metaphorically to describe a procedure for adjusting the dose of a drug. The initial dose, usually too small to produce a therapeutic response, is gradually increased over time until the desired effect is achieved or unacceptable adverse reactions appear.

TMR: trainable mentally retarded.

tolerance: a lessened susceptibility to the effects of the same dose of a drug over repeated administrations.

tonic: characterized by continuous tension. The tonic phase of a grand mal seizure is marked by boardlike rigidity.

torticollis: characterized by contracted cervical muscles resulting in a twisting of the neck and unnatural positioning of the head. A symptom of an acute dystonic reaction, an extrapyramidal syndrome associated with antipsychotic drugs.

toxic: poisonous; causing disturbance of body function or structural damage to organs and tissues.

toxic reaction: same as side effect.

trade name: a brand name protected by trademark laws which restrict use to the original copyright holder indefinitely; proprietary name, unofficial name. The trade name of a drug refers to a particular formulation of a generic drug made by a specific manufacturer.

trainable mentally retarded: an educational classification for children whose IQ's range from 25 or 35 to 50 or 55.

trauma: a wound or injury.

tremor: an involuntary trembling or shaking.

tricyclics: a category of antidepressant drugs that includes imipramine (Tofranil), amitriptyline (Elavil), and nortriptyline (Aventyl).

unilateral: affecting but one side.

untoward reaction: same as side effect.

urticaria: a skin reaction marked by patches of skin either redder or paler than the surrounding skin, usually associated with severe itching, and often caused by emotional stress or certain foods, drugs, or infections; hives.

vitamin D: a substance that greatly accelerates the absorption of calcium from the gut.

water soluble: capable of being dissolved in water.

withdrawal syndrome: characteristic symptoms associated with the withdrawal of a specific drug.

REFERENCES

Dorland's Illustrated Medical Dictionary (25th ed.). Philadelphia: Saunders, 1974.

Author Index

Subject Index

A

Abnormal Involuntary Movement Scale, 111
Absence seizures, 4, 34–35, 62, 80–81, 196, 201–202
absence status, 28
aura, 28
automatisms, 28, 196, 200, 202
description of, 27–28, 196, 201–202
drug therapy, 41–43, 82
EEG, 28, 196
tonic-clonic seizure, 42–43
Absence status, 28
Absorption, drug, 5, 16
Academic performance, 110, 147–148, 157, 183
Accidental poisoning, 3, 8, 177
Acetaphenazine (see Tindal)
Acetazolamide (see Diamox)
ACTH, 40–41, 44, 86
Acute dystonic reactions, 107–108, 117, 121, 153, 184
Acute psychosis, 145
Adolescence (see also Psychiatric disorders in adolescence), 23, 28, 34, 36, 62–63, 91
development during, 137–143
turmoil in, 140–141
Adverse drug reactions (see Side effects)
Affective disorders (see Mood disorders)
Aggressive behavior, 3, 26, 48–49, 52, 100–102, 104, 114–115, 117, 119–124, 128, 143, 155–159, 165
drug therapy, 121–124, 158–159
case study, 123–124
clinical suggestions, 159
Haldol, 121–122
Inderal, 123, 158
Lithium, 121–122, 158
Tegretol, 159
Agoraphobia, 164–166, 180
Akathisia, 107–108, 153, 184
Akinetic seizures, 33, 52
Alcohol abuse, 141, 143
Alcoholic beverages, 10, 14, 17, 175
Allegron (see Aventyl)
Allergic reaction, 10
Alprazolam, 165
American Psychiatric Association, 99–100, 119, 125, 127, 141, 145, 151